Key Concepts in Contemporary Orthodontics

Key Concepts in Contemporary Orthodontics

Edited by **Kaley Ann**

FOSTER
ACADEMICS

New Jersey

Published by Foster Academics,
61 Van Reypen Street,
Jersey City, NJ 07306, USA
www.fosteracademics.com

Key Concepts in Contemporary Orthodontics
Edited by Kaley Ann

International Standard Book Number: 978-1-63242-250-7 (Hardback)

Printed in the United States of America.

Contents

Preface

The main aim of this book is to educate learners and enhance their research focus by presenting diverse topics covering this vast field. This is an advanced book which compiles significant studies by distinguished experts in the area of analysis. This book addresses successive solutions to the challenges arising in the area of application, along with it; the book provides scope for future developments.

Orthodontics is a rapidly growing field of science as well as of medicine. The aim of this book is to provide innovative possibilities and novel ways of looking at this field. It provides key concepts in orthodontics organized under two broad sections: Orthognathic Surgery and Research. The book aims at serving the readers as a valuable means of exploration of the application of knowledge, information and answers to some orthodontic questions and topics.

It was a great honour to edit this book, though there were challenges, as it involved a lot of communication and networking between me and the editorial team. However, the end result was this all-inclusive book covering diverse themes in the field.

Finally, it is important to acknowledge the efforts of the contributors for their excellent chapters, through which a wide variety of issues have been addressed. I would also like to thank my colleagues for their valuable feedback during the making of this book.

Editor

Part 1

Orthognathic Surgery

Orthodontic-Surgical Treatment: Electromyographic and Electrognatographic Evaluation with Three Electromyographic Instruments

Giampietro Farronato, Cinzia Maspero, Lucia Giannini and Guido Galbiati
Fondazione IRCCS Ca' Granda, Ospedale Maggiore Policlinico, Milan,
Italy

1. Introduction

The introduction of electromyography in orthodontics determined the beginning of some studies about neuromuscolar system's response to physiological and pathological oral alterations and the effect of masticatory muscles on facial morphology.[1,2]

Experimental studies demonstrated that a real change in muscolar function causes morphology alterations.[1]

Several studies in literature, from Watt e Williams, who studied in 1951 the effect of masticatory bolus on mouse maxillary and mandibular development, to Avis who in 1961 showed how muscolar function was important for gonial region development, connect morpholgy and function.[3,4]

In the last years masticatory muscles response to dento-skeletal discrepancies, alterations of breathing, swelling, speech and posture, to functional therapies, implant supported therapy and prosthetic rehabilitation has been studied.[5]

The definition of occlusion changed in time and it is now not based on mechanics theory but it includes functional aspects.[6-10]

In literature different positions about the compensatory muscolar aequilibrium in skeletal discrepancies can be found.

A correct diagnosis is based not only on clinical and radiographic examination, but it is also important to analyze informations obtaining from neuromuscolar system.[2]

Knowing muscular action allows to obtain a correct diagnosis, prognosis and treatment planning and helps in avoiding failures.[2]

Electromyography allows to evaluate neuromuscolar system and equilibrium, mandibular movements alterations and the effects of orthodontic therapy on stomathognatic system.[7]

Nowadays, different kind of electromyographic instruments are available, each of them constructed following specific protocols and with different aims.

It is well known that facial growth is influenced by both genetic and extrinsic factors and that muscle function exercises an important influence both on growth and on craniofacial morphology.[11]

Orthodontic-surgical treatment was born in order to reposition the skeletal bone basis in a normal position in subjects where their position was not correct.

Modifications of the facial skeleton have consequences on all masticatory muscles, even if the majority of studies in literature is referred to masseter and temporal muscle because this muscles are easy to study with surface analysis.[12,13]

Many studies in literature have tried to highlight the effect of orthognathic surgery on neuromuscular system.

Most authors explained that a first modification of the neuromuscular system can be seen during presurgical orthodontic phase besides Precious and Skulsky showed that maximum bite force is reduced after the beginning of the fixed orthodontic therapy.[14]

Also Dean, Throckmorton and Sinn showed that patients in orthodontic-surgical treatment were able to express a minor bite force in presurgical phase if compared to the one they could express before starting therapy.[15] Thomas et al affirmed that there was a reduction of the maximum mandibular opening movement and of its movement in vertical sense before and after the orthodontic phase, connected to the same protective mechanism which explains the maximum bite force reduction.[16] Morever, during mandibular movements, there was a painful action of brackets on teeth and of orthodontics thread in soft tissues of cheek and lips, which limited the patient in executing normal movements.

Furthermore the presurgical orthodontic treatment contributed to reduce the possibility of mandibular movements and the consequent reduction of occlusal contacts, increasing interferences between dental elements with reduction of mandibular excursion.[17-21]

Many studies analyzed the modifications consequent to a surgical reposition of bone basis.

Finn, Throckmorton, Bell and Legan did not show an increase of the maximum muscular force post surgical of muscular advancement and maxillary retroposition.[22]

Also Van den Braber et al affirmed that oral function is not influenced by mandibular advancement surgery.[23] On the contrary round Athanasiou had discovered that surgical correction of maxillary prognathism increased the intensity of occlusal contacts and hypothesized that such harmonization of the dentofacial skeleton would influence the neuromuscular system.[24] Kobayashi et al affirmed that the steadiness of the masticatory rhythm is improved by orthognathic surgery in subjects with mandibular prognathism.[25]

A Tatsumi et al study has proved that, after the surgical orthodontic treatment, an aesthetic improvement, a reduction of the duration of the masticatory cycle and an improvement of the activity of masticatory muscles are obtained.[26] These advantages suggest that patients who undergo this operation gain a functional readjustment in post-surgical phase Proffit reported a maximum bite force increase in some patients in post-surgical phase. Unfortunately, this increase was not an improvement compared to the beginning of the therapy, but a return to initial conditions before starting orthodontic therapy.

These changes underwent a huge variability, due to the different sensibility of patients on dental, muscular and articulation level. Besides, to explain the obtained results, the patient's will and emotional stress were probably more important than muscular advantages and biomechanics.

The majority of studies have analyzed only a single phase of the treatment.

The aim of this work consists in the evaluation of the neuromuscular functionality and mandibular kinesiology in 100 patients undergoing orthodontic surgical treatment.

Values obtained analyzing masticatory muscles in patients with important skeletal discrepancies using three different kind of electromyographic instruments were compared.

Orthodontic-Surgical Treatment: Electromyographic and Electrognatographic Evaluation with Three
Electromyographic Instruments

5

2. Material and methods

Study group

All patients during the orthognathic surgery treatment at the Orthodontic Section of the department of Surgical, Reconstructive and Diagnostic Sciences have been submitted to classical instrumental exams, clinical and radiographic, and also periodically to an electromyographic and electrokinesiographic evaluation.

The analyzed sample is composed of 100 patients [44 men and 56 women] at the end of growth.

Criteria followed in selecting patients were:
-   adult age
-   the presence of a dento-skeletal discrepancy
-   the necessity of a combined orthodontic-surgical treatment

The three criteria had to coexist at the same time.

The electromiographic and the kinesiographic examination have been performed on orthodontic-surgical patients:
-   during the first visit
-   before the start of the orthodontic therapy
-   during the presurgical phase of orthodontic bimonthly
-   every month from three months before the surgical operation to three months after
-   the day before the surgical operation
-   during the intermaxillary fixation
-   at the removal of the fixation
-   during post-surgical orthodontic phase with the same terms (times) of pre-surgical orthodontic phase.
-   at the removal of surgical bite
-   at the end of the treatment
-   during follow up

In every phase, patients executed two electromyographic examinations through two different electromyograms.

Before every tests clinicans asked patients if they had dental or muscolar pain in order to avoid errors.

The electromyographic instruments used in the work were the electromiography Freely [De Gotzen – Legnano - Italia], the electromiography and electrognatography K6-I EMG [Myotronics – Tukwila WA – USA] and the electromiography and electrognatography Biopak [Bioresearch Associate -USA].

The muscles considered have been the anterior temporal muscle and the masseter muscle.

In order to compare the data versus the healthy population, a control group has been settled. This group consists of patients in adult age, skeletal class I, with absence of temporal-mandibular problems and absence of a previous orthodontic or a combined orthodontic-surgical treatment.

Finally a statistic test evaluation has been performed with t test and ANOVA test.

Methods

The muscles considered in the electromyographic evaluation have been:
-   the anterior temporal muscle
-   the masseter muscle in its superficial component

- The patient was in a special totally undisturbed and noiseless room. He sat on a rigid stool with an adjustable height, so to have the angle between thigh and leg of 90° (degrees).

The legs were parallel to the floor, the back upright and the gaze beyond the horizon.

Head was in natural head position.

After skin cleaning with a wad soaked in Neoxinal (clorexidina 0,5% in hydroalcoholic solution with no less than 70% of alcohol) to reduce forehead impedance and facilitate adhesiveness, electrodes were positioned.

The electrodes position was the same for both the equipments and unmodified with the use of either equipment.

The electrodes were disposable and bipolar, Duo Trade Silver/ Silver Chloride previously gelled. The interpolar distance was of 21±1 mm, each pole was circular, 10 mm in diameter.

The bipolar electrodes were positioned according to the following procedure:

- for the masseter muscle: the operator, behind a seated subject, palpates the belly of the muscle while the patient clenches his teeth. To position the bipolar electrode parallel to the muscle fibres, the line connecting the commissura labiorum oris with the tragum is ideally drawn as well as the line connecting the the the lateral part of eye and gonion.

The position of the electrode makes the superior pole in the intersection point between the two lines and its major axis is along the esocanto-goniac line.

- for the temporal muscle: the muscle is palpated while clenching thus localizing the major axis of the zygomatic process of the frontal bone.

The bipolar electrode is positioned along the line parallel to this process passing about a transverse finger posteriorly and superiorly to it; this way the electrode will be parallel to the muscle fibres and positioned more or less superficially in comparison with the frontoparietal suture.

A grounding electrode (monopolar) is positioned on a silent muscular area of the forehead.

Such electrode may be positioned on the volar surface of the forearm, considered a possible silent area. The electromyographic instrument utilises such electrode as a reference eliminating part of all background noises. So, it can be considered a first filter to abolish interferences.

The tests with the two instruments are executed consecutively without taking off electrodes.

An average of data collected by each patient was then done at every therapeutic phase.

3. Results

At the beginning of the treatment the patients present a compensatory equilibrium to malocclusion. During presurgical orthodontic phase electromyographic and electrognatographic values become worse and they continue worsening after surgical intervention. They improve in post surgical orthodontic phase.

After the removal of the orthodontic appliance, electromyographic values improve until they reach optimal values. Mandibular movement rehabilitation is satisfactory and constant also if it needs more time than muscular rehabilitation. At the end of the treatment maximum mandibular opening is still less than the preoperatory one. (fig. 1-14)

The three instruments have been planned through different principles, they are based on different ideas and they have different aims.

The different types does not avoid the possibility to obtain complementary data, not even in numeric values, but in their meaning. (fig. 15-21)

Orthodontic-Surgical Treatment: Electromyographic and Electrognatographic Evaluation with Three
Electromyographic Instruments

7

Data obtained from all instruments gives to the clinicians the same information, also if they are expressed in different ways.

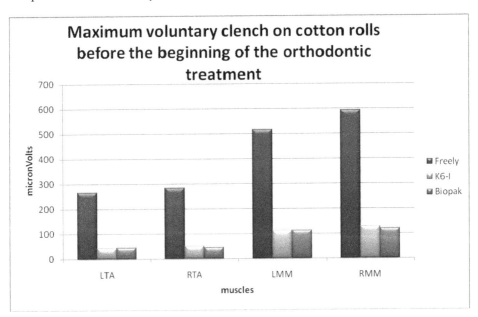

Fig. 1.

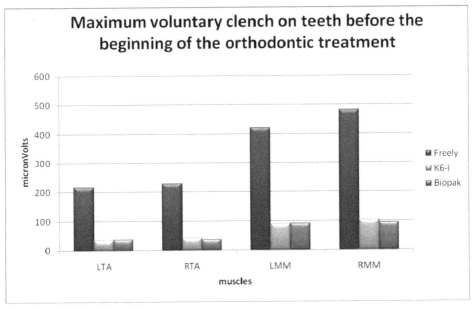

Fig. 2.

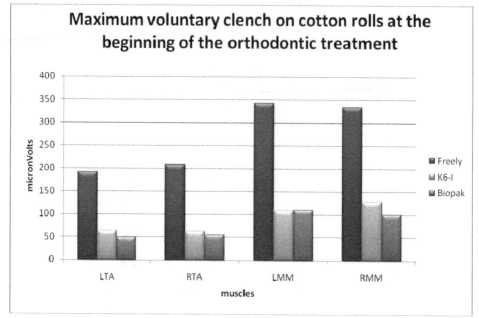

Fig. 3.

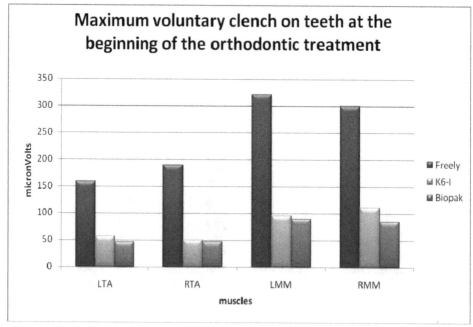

Fig. 4.

Orthodontic-Surgical Treatment: Electromyographic and Electrognatographic Evaluation with Three
Electromyographic Instruments

9

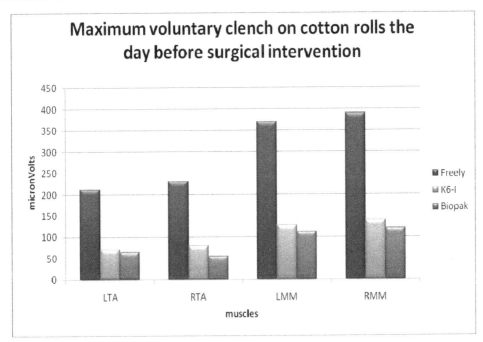

Fig. 5.

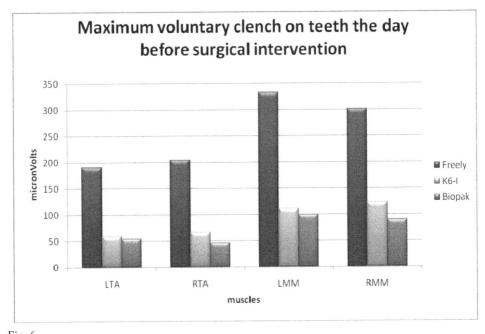

Fig. 6.

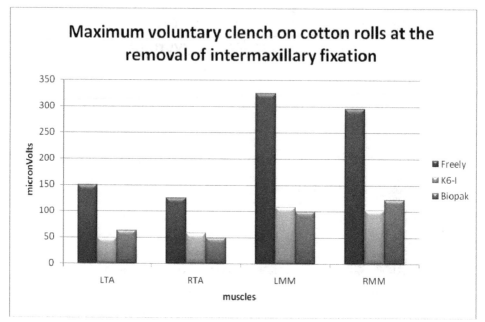

Fig. 7.

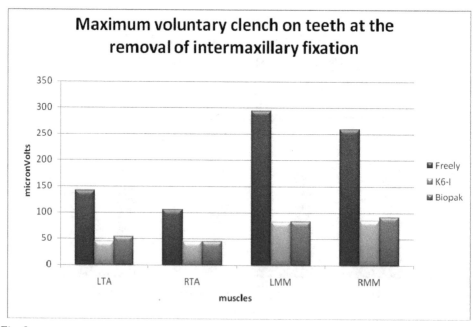

Fig. 8.

Orthodontic-Surgical Treatment: Electromyographic and Electrognatographic Evaluation with Three
Electromyographic Instruments

11

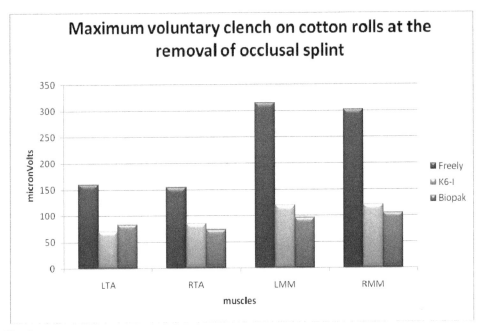

Fig. 9.

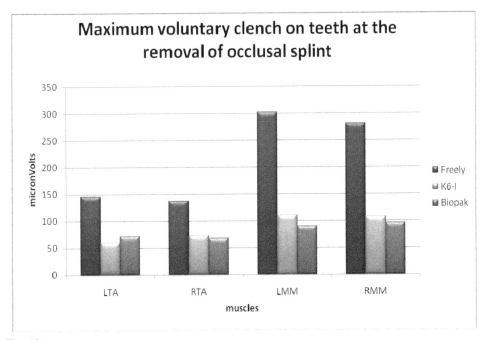

Fig. 10.

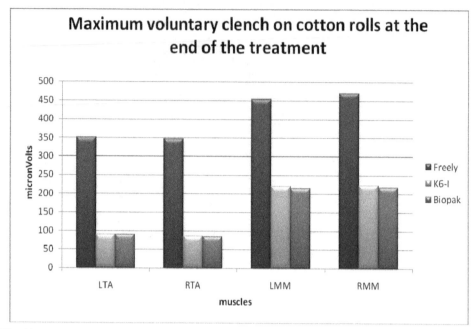

Fig. 11.

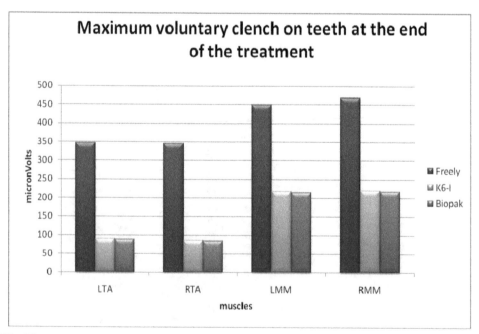

Fig. 12.

Orthodontic-Surgical Treatment: Electromyographic and Electrognatographic Evaluation with Three
Electromyographic Instruments

13

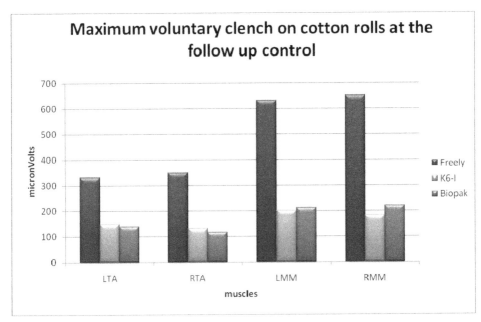

Fig. 13.

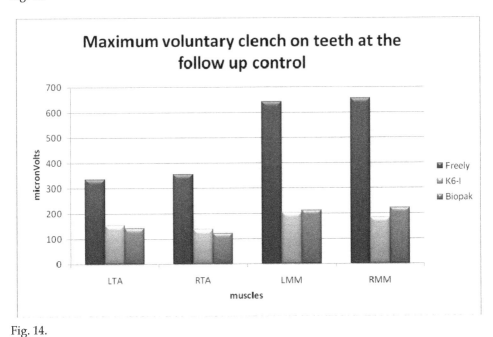

Fig. 14.

Fig. 1-14. Maximum voluntary clench on cotton rolls and on teeth during the different phases of the treatment.

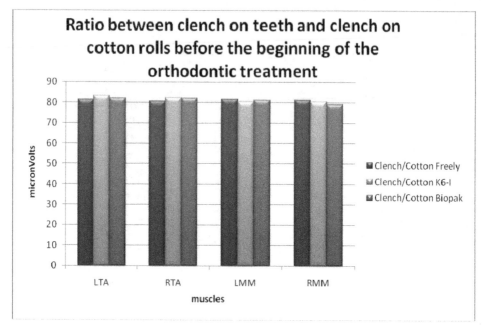

Fig. 15.

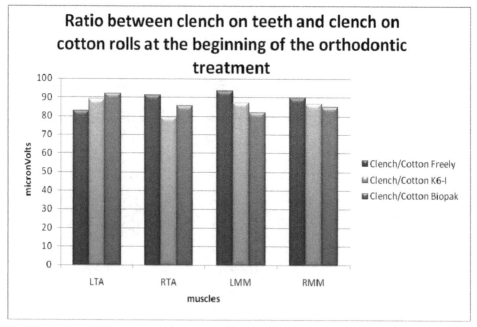

Fig. 16.

Orthodontic-Surgical Treatment: Electromyographic and Electrognatographic Evaluation with Three
Electromyographic Instruments

15

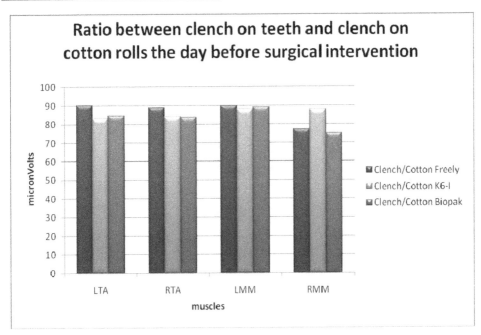

Fig. 17.

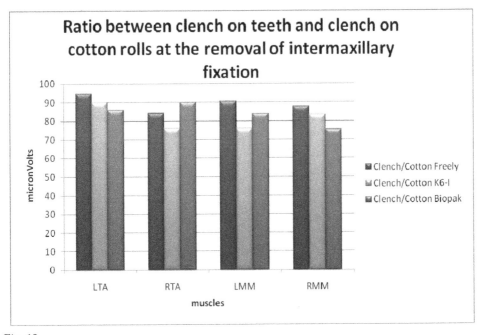

Fig. 18.

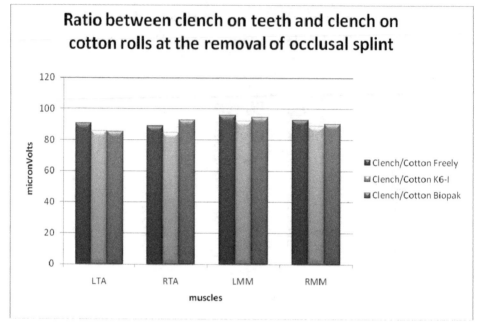

Fig. 19.

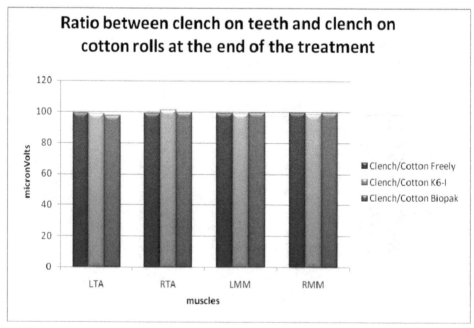

Fig. 20.

Orthodontic-Surgical Treatment: Electromyographic and Electrognatographic Evaluation with Three
Electromyographic Instruments

17

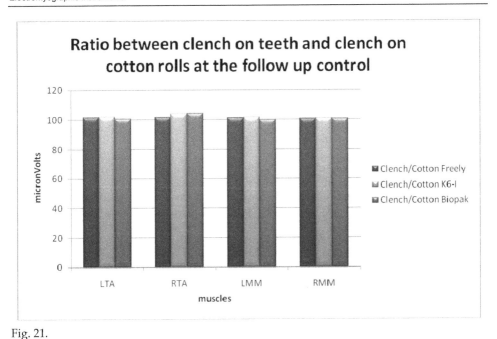

Fig. 21.

Fig. 15-21. Ratio between maximum voluntary clench on cotton rolls and on teeth during the different phases of the treatment.

4. Discussion

The instruments have been planned through different principles, they are based on different ideas and they have different aims.

The protocol studied for Freely by Ferrario et al has been organized in order to obtain the maximum of reproducibility because it is based on a standardized methods which allows to evaluate real percent data.[6]

Following this protocol, micronVolt in maximum voluntary clench on teeth and on cotton rolls were not considered in order to avoid false evaluations.[6]

Besides, this protocol consists in evaluating tests executed in clench on teeth and in comparing them with the ones executed on cotton rolls, in order to obtain percent data with a higher degree of reliability because of the override of every kind of interference due to a non correct position in electrodes or to other external variables.

K6-I electromyograph was projected based on different principles and it does not do this calculation. Besides, ratio between maximum voluntary clenac on teeth and on cotton rolls have been calculated manually in order to obtain data comparable with Freely.

Moreover, the instruments are calibrated in different way and they use different amplifiers and signal filters.

Besides, comparing micronVolt values registered on both instruments in the same time, huge differences can be underlined, but comparing their percent values obtained from clench/cotton ratio similar data can be obtained.

This indicate that the micronVolt muscle activity is different from the two instruments but their percent values are similar and both electromyographs can be overlapped.

Expecially, in this study in patients in orthodontic-surgical therapy, values obtained by the instruments are more similar in the phases which preceed the orthodontic surgical therapy and at the end of the treatment.

In the immediate postsurgical phase, patients have an instable occlusion and there is a lower reproducibility of the measurements.

Lots of differences between skeletal class II and skeletal class III patients have been evidenced by the analysis of the data obtained.

The IMPACT index, which underlines the muscular force expression in time, is definitely major in skeletal class II patients than in skeletal class III patients almost in all treatment phases.

Such difference is statistically significative. Only at the end of the treatment does not a statistically significative difference between the different groups persist.

The activity of the four muscular fasciae, expressed in micronVolt, is definitely major in skeletal class II than in skeletal class III subjects at the beginning of the treatment.

This difference, statistically significative, tends to disappear in the successive phases.

These results have been obtained both on the exercises with cotton rolls between the arches and in clench, with both the electromyographic systems.

As regards mandibular kinesiology, the maximum mandibular opening movement is wider in skeletal class III patients in all the treatment phases, except for the end of the therapy.

The protrusive movement is always major in skeletal class II patients. This gap is reduced at the end of the therapy, but it does persist.

Statistically significative differences about right and left lateral movements have not been evidenced.

By a comparison of the temporal muscle PERCENT OVERLAPPING COEFFICIENT [POC] index it has been underlined that in the initial phases the muscular activity presents a reduced neuromuscular equilibrium. Skeletal class II patients are particularly uncompensated at the beginning of the treatment. After the start of the orthodontic therapy the POC index improves but the value, which isn't included in the physiological range, is constant up to the surgical operation. In the last part of the surgical orthodontic treatment the POC index improves and at the end of the treatment it is included in the physiological range. Skeletal class III patients present in the pre-surgical phases values close to the physiologic limit and improve only at the end of the treatment. Values are physiologic at the end of the treatment.

Skeletal class II patients present a major harmony in the temporal muscle activity compared with skeletal class III patients. The masseter muscle POC index presents a light reduction of the overriding range of the muscular activity after the appliance cementing. This value improves up to the end of the treatment, when the POC index is similar in all skeletal class.

As regards POC medium progressive improvement of the value between the first acquisition made at the beginning of the treatment until the end of the fix orthodontic therapy can be noticed.

Class II patients are more overriding than class III patients at the beginning of treatment. At the end of treatment POC values underline a sufficient neuro-muscular equilibrium, yet there is a difference of about two points of percentage between the classes (the index is slightly better for class II patients).

The progressive improvement of POC indexes in all classes shows that orthodontic treatment tends to develop a major equilibrium among different muscular activities.

As regards POC index a similar progress to skeletal class II and III patients has been noticed even in small samples, hence the insertion of the value of skeletal class I patients in the relative figures.

Orthodontic-Surgical Treatment: Electromyographic and Electrognatographic Evaluation with Three
Electromyographic Instruments

19

TORS index shows similar values in skeletal class II and III patients, without the attainment performed at the beginning of the treatment; data remain higher than the normal value [considered equal to 10%] during the period of the orthodontic treatment, at the end of the treatment the TORS value is nearly normal.

The ASIMMETRY index which shows the side of prevalence has an opposite course between the two classes, that is, while for class III patients it diminishes up to the attainment performed in the final part of the orthodontic post-surgical treatment where it starts to increase again, class II patients have an opposite response, nevertheless values are still quite normal.

About the index of TORQUE, class II patients tend to have an occlusal prior centre of mass [negative value], in order to become positive in post-surgical attainments and to arrange themselves close to zero at the end of the treatment. In class III patients the index always remains positive [posterior contact] and it always remains in the range of normality; at the end of the treatment the value is close to zero.

TORQUE index has an alternating course in both classes, its values are quite normal.

The ability in developing force in time in the test on cotton rolls shows a course in part superposable between the two skeletal classes, the decrease of the force up to the level of the attainments performed after the beginning of the orthodontic therapy and after the surgical operation it remains constant, in order get back to the previous values at the end of the treatment. Also the course of the IMPACT in the test of the greatest clench shows a similar response, but not completely superposable between two skeletal classes; nevertheless the decreases of the value of IMPACT up to the level of the surgical operation are still confirmed.

The IMPACT values %*sec highlighted by the two classes show a partial superposable course, with the exclusion of the attainment performed after the beginning of the orthodontic therapy in class II patients where the value tends to diminish, while it increases in class III patients. Finally all the values are quite normal [100 ± 15%*sec] but for the attainment performed after the period of intermaxillary block. At the end of the treatment values are slightly inferior than 100%*sec.

Observing more data of class II and III patients, it has to be noticed that the first group develops a minor muscular activity in comparison to the second group, nevertheless in the other levels class II patients develop a major electric energy, during all the orthodontic fixed treatment, the same observations can be noticed for IMPACT indexes µV*sec. This factual information could be connected to the reduced number of subjects who have an attainment in the initial phase, and it could be the same for attainments performed at the end of the treatment. Considering the afore said things and observing the index of medium POC, there's to notice that even if on the one hand skeletal class III develop a major clench force, it is always true that these result balance than class II patients [medium POC class II patients =80%; class III patients=78%] and the program connected to the electromyography Freely results more important and bases itself on data got from formulas instead from relative values.

Lots of differences between open and deep skeletal bite patients have been underlined by the analysis of the electromyographic data obtained at the beginning of the treatment.

The impact value and muscular activity in micronVolt analysis shows a major muscle activity in deep bite patients than in deep bite ones.

These results have been obtained with both the electromiographic systems.

The following authors too proved that high angle cases were associated with weaker musculature than low angle patients: Möller (1966), Sassouni (1969), Ingerval et al (1974), Bakke (1991), Kayukawa (1992), Farronato (1992) and Bong Kuen Cha (2007). [27-33]

Ahlgren et al. (1973, 1985) proved a positively correlation between the mandibular plane angle (SNGoMe) and the temporal muscle activity (TMA).[34,35] Moller and Ingervall obtained opposite results.[36,37]

Ueda et al (1998) proved that vertical craniofacial morphology is positively correlated with temporal muscle activity (TMA) and negative correlated with masseter muscle activity (MMA).[11]

Fogle et al. (1995) obtained opposite results. They proved that a correlation between craniofacial morphology and masticatory function doesn't exist. The only correlation is between muscle function and patients age.[38] The differences existing between the two groups at the beginning of the treatment, statistically significative, tend to disappear at the removal of the fix orthodontic appliance confirming the orthodontic surgical treatment's corrective role in according to Santoro's study.[39]

Furthermore, before the starting of the fix orthodontic therapy, patients present a compensatory equilibrium to disgnatia. During successive phases electromyographic and electrognatographic continue worsening according to Oliver et al (1985), Proffith et al (1989), Brown et al (1991) and Thomas et al (1995). They improve in post surgical orthodontic phase only.[40-43]

At the end of the orthodontic surgical treatment electromyographic values improve and reach optimal values.

Mandibular movement rehabilitation needs more time than the muscular one even if it is satisfactory and constant too.

At the end of the treatment maximum mandibular opening is still less than the preoperatory one.

No statistically significative differences between the two groups have been highlighted about mandibular kinesiology.

5. Conclusion

This study confirms that the functional rehabilitation in patients in orthodontic-surgical treatment occurs in a good way and in a good time.

The functional evaluation in patients during orthodontic-surgical therapy is an important element to reduce as much as possible a incorrect neuromuscular activity that can cause a relapse; it also helps clinicians to follow treatment phases and to control the results obtained.

6. References

[1] Serrao G. Relation between vertical facial morphology and jaw muscle activity in healthy young man. Prog Orthod 2003;4:45-51.

[2] Farronato G. Aesthetic in Ortodontic surgery. Rivista Italiana di chirurgia maxillo-facciale 2003;14(3):123-6.

[3] Avis V. The significance of the angle of the mandible: an experimental and comparative study. Am J Phys Anthropol 1961;19:55-61.

[4] Watt DG. The effects of the physical consistency of food on the growth and development of the mandible and the maxilla of the rat. Am J Orthod 1951;37(12):895-928.

Orthodontic-Surgical Treatment: Electromyographic and Electrognatographic Evaluation with Three
Electromyographic Instruments

21

[5] Ferrario VF. The effects of a single intercuspal interference on electromyographic characteristics of human masticatory muscles during maximal voluntary teeth clenching. J Craniomandib Pract 1999;17:184-8.

[6] Ferrario VF. The use of surface electromyography as a tool in differentiating temporomandibular disorders from neck disorders. Man Ther 2007;12(4):372-9.

[7] Jankelson B. Kinesiometrik instrumentation: a new technology. JADA 1975;90:834-40.

[8] Jankelson B. The physiology of the sthomatognatic system. JADA 1953;46:375-86.

[9] Jankelson. Physiological aspects of masticatory muscle stimulation the myomonitor. Quintessence Int Dent Dig 1972;3(12):57-62.

[10] Jankelson B. The intherited methodology of occlusion. Calif Dent Ass meeting San Francisco 1976;10:1-3.

[11] Ueda HM, Ishizuda Y, Miyamoto N, Morimoto N, Tanne K: Relationship between masticatory muscle activity and vertical craniofacial morphology. Angle Orthod 68:233-238,1998.

[12] Sforza C, Peretta R,Grandi G, Ferronato G,Ferrario VF. Soft Tissue Facial Planes and Masticatory Muscle Function in Skeletal Class III Patients Before and After Orthognathic Surgery Treatment. J Oral Maxillofac Surg 66:691-698,2008.

[13] Throckmorton GS, Ellis E III, Bushang PH. Morphologic and biomechanical correlates with maximum bite forces in orthognathicsurgery patients. J Oral Maxillofac Surg 58:515,2000.

[14] Precious DS, Goodday RH, Bourget L, Skulsky FG. Pterygoid plate fracture in Le Fort I osteotomy with and without pterygoid chisel: a computed tomography scan evaluation of 58 patients. J Oral Maxillofac Surg 51(2):151-3,1983.

[15] Dean JS, Throckmorton GS, Ellis E 3rd, Sinn DP. A preliminary study of maximum voluntary bite force and jaw muscle efficiency in pre-orthognathic surgery patients.J Oral Maxillofac Surg 50(12):1284-8,1992.

[16] Thomas GP, Throckmorton GS, Ellis E III, Sinn DP. The effects of orthodontic treatment on isometric bite forces and mandibular motion in patients before orthognathic surgery. J Oral Maxillofac Surg 53:673–678,1995.

[17] Proffit WR, Turvey TA, Fields HW, Phillips C. The effect of orthognathic surgery on occlusal force. J Oral Maxillofac Surg 47:457–463,1989.

[18] Braun S, Bantleon HP, Hnat WP, Freudenthaler JW, Marcotte MR, Johnson BE. A study of bite force. Part 2. Relationship to various cephalometric measurements. Angle Orthod 65:373–377,1994.

[19] Bertelè GP: Trattamento ortodontico-chirurgico. Dental Cadmos 4:13,1989.

[20] Farronato G, Maspero C, Giannini L, Farronato D. Occlusal splint guides for presurgical orthodontic treatment. Journal of clinical orthodontics 9:508-12,2008.

[21] Farronato G, Maspero C, Paini L, Farronato D. Sistematica di programmazione ortodontica-pre chirurgica. Mondo Ortodontico 3:197-202,2004.

[22] Finn RA, Throckmorton GS, Bell WH, Legan HL. Biomechanical considerations in the surgical correction of mandibular deficiency.correction of mandibular deficiency. J Oral Surg 38:257–263,1980.

[23] Van den Braber W, Van der Bilt A, Van der Glas H, Rosenberg T, Koole R. The influence of mandibular advancement surgery on oral function in retrognathic patients: a 5-year follow-up study. J Oral Maxillofac Surg 64(8):1237-40,2006.

[24] Athanasiou AE, Toutountzakis N, Mavreas D, Ritzau M, Wenzel A. Alterations of hyoid bone position and pharyngeal depth and their relationship after surgical

correction of mandibular prognathism. Am J Orthod Dentofacial Orthop 100(3):259-65,1991.

[25] Kobayashi T, Honma K, Shingaki S, Nakajima T: Changes in masticatory function after orthognathic treatment in patients with mandibular prognathism 39(4):260-5,2001.

[26] Tatsumi H, Takada K, Hiraki T, Sakuda M, Minami K, Mori Y, Sugahara T, Sakuda M. A cephalometric electromyographic and kinesiographic appraisal of a patient with mandibular prognathism and anterior openbite malocclusion before and after surgical orthodontic therapy a case report. Osaka Daigaku Shigaku Zasshi 35(2):618-32,1990.

[27] Möller E. The chewing apparatus. Acta Physiol 1966; 69: 571-4.

[28] Ingervall B, Thilander B. Relation between facial morphology and activity of the masticatory muscles. J Oral Rehabil 1974; 1: 131–147.

[29] Bakke M, Michler L. Temporalis and masseter muscle activity in patients with anterior open bite and craniomandibular disorders. Scand J Dent Res 1991 Jun; 99(3): 219-28.

[30] Kayukawa. Malocclusion and masticatory muscle activity: a comparison of your types of malocclusion. J Clin Pediatr Dent 1992; 16(3): 162-77.

[31] Farronato G, Giannì AB, Bianchini R. Problematiche ortognatodontiche funzionali ed open-bite dentario contributo elettromiografico (emg) ed elettrognatografico (egg). Ortognatodonzia Italiana 1992; 3(1):307-321.

[32] Bong K.C, Chun-Hi K, Seung-Hak B. Skeletal Sagittal and Vertical Facial Types and Electromyographic Activity of the Masticatory Muscle. Angle Orthodontist 2007: 77(3): 463-470.

[33] Sassouni V. A classification of skeletal facial types. Am J Orthod 1969; 55: 109-114.

[34] Ahlgren JG, Ingervall BF, Thilander BL. Muscle activity in normal and postnormal occlusion. Am J Orthod. 1973;64: 445–456.

[35] Ahlgren J, Sonesson B, Blitz M. An electromyographic analysis of the temporalis function of normal occlusion. Am J Orthod 1985;87:230–239.

[36] Ingervall B. Facial morphology and activity of temporal and lip muscles during swallowing and chewing. Angle Orthod 1976; 46: 372–380.

[37] Möller E. The chewing apparatus. Acta Physiol 1966; 69: 571-4.

[38] Fogle LL, Glaros AG. Contributions of facial morphology age and gender to EMG activity under biting and resting conditions a canonical correlation analysis. J Dent Res 1995; 74: 1496–1500.

[39] Santoro F, Maiorana C. Il trattamento ortodontico-chirurgico delle disgnazie. Milano: Ariesdue; 1998.

[40] Thomas GP, Throckmorton GS, Ellis E III, Sinn DP. The effects of orthodontic treatment on isometric bite forces and mandibular motion in patients before orthognathic surgery. J Oral Maxillofac Surg 1995; 53: 673–678.

[41] Proffit WR, Turvey TA, Fields HW, Phillips C. The effect of orthognathic surgery on occlusal force. J Oral Maxillofac Surg 1989; 47: 457–463.

[42] Brown DF, Moerenhout RG. The pain experience and psychological adjustment to orthodontic treatment of preadolescents, adolescents and adults. Am J Orthod Dentofac Orthop 1991; 100: 349-56.

[43] Oliver RG, Knapman YM. At Attitudes to orthodontic treatment. Br J Orthod 1985; 12: 179-88.

2

Orthodontic Contribution to Orthognathic Surgery Cases

Nikolaos Topouzelis

Aristotle University of Thessaloniki, Dental School
Greece

1. Introduction

Skeletal malocclusion (dysgnathia) is defined as the congenital or acquired abnormal position or morphology of one or both jaws. There might be symmetry or asymmetry with disruption of the maxillomandibular relationship or the relationship of the jaws to the skull base combined with malocclusion or joint disruption. The main treatment objectives for serious skeletal malocclusions are aesthetic, functional and psychological rehabilitation. For this kind of cases these goals may be achieved. The orthodontist can move teeth and alveoli but this has no substantial impact on the adult basal jaw bone. The main orthodontist's task is teeth alignment. The oral & maxilofacial surgeon is responsible for the surgical correction of jaws and their associated structures. Generally speaking, the diagnosis and treatment plan of orthognathic cases require a systematic team approach. Although team member composition may differ depending on conditions at any given time, an ideal team should include an orthodontist, a maxillofacial surgeon, a phychiatrist or a clinical phychologist, a prosthetologist and a specialised dental technician. Orthognathic surgery involves risks and this is why we need to proceed with it only after careful planning. It is particularly important to understand the patient's view; this establishes trust and communication and helps achieve high quality results.

The management protocol for dentofacial abnormalities, treated through the cooperation of orthodontics and orthognathic surgery involves taking detailed medical and dental history of the patient, clinical examination, casts analysis, photographs, radiographs analysis (leading to diagnosis and treatment plan), presurgical orthodontics, actual surgery and post-surgical orthodontics.

2. Medical history

Taking a comprehensive medical history is of the utmost importance. Most orthognathic patients are young individuals and their health normally allows then to undergo general anaesthesia and extensive surgery. However, there are specific disorders, such as blood diseases (coagulation disorders), hormonal disorders, heart diseases, allergies, rheumatic diseases, respiratory diseases (sleep apneoa), which require special treatment (Harris & Hunt, 2008).

Very serious facial disproportions might be associated with systemic diseases, such as acromegaly (Class III cases) or chronic juvenile arthrities and muscular dystrophy (Class II cases with open bite). Such medical problems complicate orthognathic treatment and may lead to a generally unstable result if not sufficiently controlled. Furthermore, patients' psychological assessment is essential so as to ensure that their expectations are realistic. Besides, the case of dysmorphobia should be examined, because such patients are totally unsuitable for orthognathic treatment, as they are bound to be disappointed by the result (Winchester & Young, 2007).

3. Dental history

When taking the patient's dental history, existing teeth should be recorded and any caries or periodontal problems identified and treated before orthodontic treatment and orthognathic surgery, in coooperation with specialised dentists. However, there might be problems such as missing teeth which would be better treated after orthognathic surgery. Orthodontic intra-oral examination must include: a) assessment of static and functional occlusion and dental base relationships in the three spatial dimensions. It is important to check and record if there are extreme lateral or protrusive mandibular movements along the mandible elevation path, in cases of anterior or posterior cross-bite and in cases of disruption of the relationship between the upper and lower midline or the relationship between the upper and lower midlline the midline of the face; b) the presence of tooth spacing or crowding in relation to possible tooth size or morphology disorders; c) the presence of tooth displacement or rotation; d) the presence of anterior teeth inclination, since upper incisors become apparent when they are labially inclined, while lower incisors become apparent in patients with Class III skeletal dyscrepancy when these teeth are lingually inclined; e) checking incisal overbite and overjet. In cases of open bite, it should be checked whether there is a step at the occlusal plane in the upper arch and the anterior teeth are positioned higher than the lower ones; f) occlusal plane disorders, which are checked in the anteroposterior and vertical dimensions using the curve of Spee and in the transverse dimension using the curve of Wilson, which assesses the buccal-lingual position of the occlusal surface of posterior upper and lower teeth; g) the morphology of the dental arches and the palate. In cleft cases, a careful analysis of their type and extension is necessary as well as an examination of bone deficits that require grafts (Harris & Hunt, 2008); h) tongue assessment. A sizeable tongue (macroglossia) may lead to dental and skeletal problems and undermine the stability of the outcome of the orthodontic and orthognathic treatment; it may also cause problems with mastication, speech and breathing; i) examination of tonsil size, since their excessive size may cause respiratory problems; j) recording problems related to masticatory muscles and the temporomandibular joint, so that if related problems appear after treatment, there will be no confusion as to whether they preexisted or not; if possible, such problems should be dealt with before treatment starts. It is important to advise patients to ensure they fully comprehend that orthognathic surgery takes place so as to correct dento-mandibular disorders and its impact on a preexisting temporomandibular dysfunction is unpredictable; in fact the problem may be exacerbated postoperatively (Onizawa et al., 1995).

4. Clinical examination of the face

Clinical examination in regard to facial aesthetics and symmetry is more successful when the patient is sitting comfortably, with the horizontal Frankfurt plane parallel to the ground or in a normal position, with the dental arches in central occlusion and the lips totally relaxed. The aim of the clinical examination, in combination with cephalometric radiography and photographs is to recognise whether the maxilla, the mandible or both jaws are pathological and to note other important facial features.

4.1 Frontal clinical examination

The frontal facial view is what the patient sees in the mirror and it is also what is usually seen by other people in personal interaction. This is why this view is of particular significance. Numerous major facial parameters can be assessed in frontal view in regard to both the vertical and the transverse dimension. Maximum facial width should be assessed through the inter-zygomatic width. The ratio of facial height to width should be 1.3:1 for women and 1.35:1 for men (Fig. 1). Another quite significant measurement is the bigonial width, which should be around 30% shorter than the bizygomatic width (Fig. 1). However, according to current beauty standards, faces where the bigonial width is longer than normal are preferred (Winchester & Young, 2007). The conventional way to assess the vertical dimension of the face is to ensure that there are three equal vertical parts (Fig. 1). The upper part is between the hairline and the eyebrows, the middle part between the eyebrows and the base of the nose and the lower part from the base of the nose to the gnathion. It is important to examine if the vertical height of the three parts is excessive or deficient, in particular regarding the middle third that entails the maxilla and the lower third that entails the mandible (Sarver et al., 2003). In the lower facial third, the ratio of the upper lip height to the lower lip and chin height should be 1:2 (Fig. 1). A pronounced labiomental fold may indicate a reduced anterior facial height, while a shallow fold an increased height.

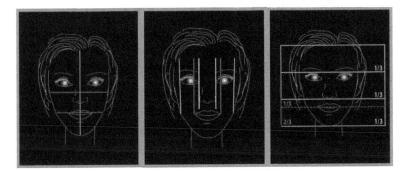

Fig. 1. Facial proportions

When assessing the transverse dimension of the face, it is important to initially note any asymmetry of the middle or lower third of the face. When the upper or lower dental midlines of a patient do not coincide or do not agree with the skeletal midlines (Fig. 9) differential diagnosis is essential in order to follow the right treatment.

The nose is a central structure of the face and plays a particularly important role during clinical examination. Traditionally, among Caucasians, it was acceptable that the alar base width as measured from the lateral aspects of the alar cartilages of the nose, should be more or less equal to the inter-canthal distance, as measured between the medial canthi of the eyes (Fig. 1). This assessment is important when maxillary impaction is planned (Harris & Hunt, 2008). The width of the mouth should be more or less equal to the distance between the medial borders of the iris (Fig. 1). Similarly, the width of the mandible at the level of the gonion should be more or less equal to the distance between the lateral canthi of the eyes (Sarver et al., 2003).

Dentolabial relationships play an important role in facial aesthetics and they should be assessed at a resting position as well as in function while the patient is smiling. The visible part of the teeth and gingivae under the upper lip is important when making a decision concerning maxillary depression or lower maxillary repositioning. At rest, 2-3 mm of the incisors should be visible. Higher figures, up to 5 mm, have also been proposed (Arnett & Bermann, 1993a, 1993b) following the rationale that more exposure of the teeth is acceptable among women than among men. When laughing, the whole of the central incisor up to the level of marginal gingivae should be visible or even including 1-2 mm of the attached gingivae. More extensive exposure of the attached gums is more acceptable among women than among men. (Guariglia & Ronchi, 2005).

4.2 Profile clinical examination

When examining the face from its side view, what is first reviewed are, again, the previously referred vertical proportions (Fig. 2) and any balance and harmony problems in the sagittal dimension.

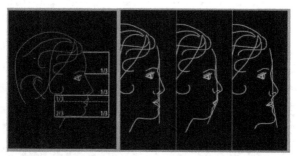

Fig. 2. Vertical proportions and reference lines for facial profile assessment

The nose and its features are also examined because nasal appearance may often undergo related and anatomical alterations in many osteotomies. So, in a Le Fort I osteotomy, maxillary impaction will tend to elevate the tip of the nose and restrict the nasal hump. What should also be assessed is the nasolabial angle; higher values tend to be more acceptable among women, while lower values among men. An acute nasolabial angle may be associated with maxillary hypoplasia and, therefore, may be improved with surgical maxillary protrusion. Controlling maxillary and mandibular protrusion or retrusion is assessed with two vertical lines. The first line goes through the most prominent part of the forehead (Fig. 2) and the second line goes through the soft tissue nasion. In a harmonious face, the end of the lips should touch the first line while maxillary soft tissues should be about 2-3 mm anterior to the second line and the chin should be 2 mm posterior to the second line (Winchester & Young, 2007).

In cases of sagittal disorder of the maxillomandibular relation, differential clinical aetiology diagnosis may become apparent in Class III cases, by filling the upper lip with soft wax or cotton (Fig. 3) until the relationship between the lips and the facial profile approximates what is considered normal. Similarly, surgical correction of a retruded mandible may be represented by asking the patient to slide the mandible forward.

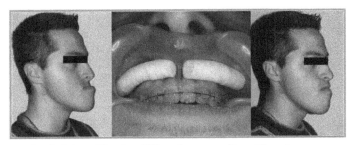

Fig. 3. Change in the facial profile after filling the upper lip with cotton

The submental region should be examined to check for the presence of excessive fat or a double-chin appearance, which is often associated with a short neck. Sometimes, mandibular set back may enhance this subcutaneous tissue deposit. This may be a contra-indication for mandibular set back or may make liposuction or plastic surgery necessary. However, among young patients, the submental region is usually spontaneously contoured after the operation.

5. Laboratory examinations

5.1 Casts
Casts should represent all the teeth that are present, the alveolar processes, the frenulums and the grooves (gingivolabial, gingivo-buccal, gingivolingual). The bases of the casts are trimmed in the intercuspal or central occlusion position, with the help of the corresponding bite records. The casts provide the best data for the assessment of dental problems and static occlusion. Initially they are examined separately in regard to arch shape (parabolic, triangular, square), rotations, deviations and ectopic and infraoccluded teeth. Crowding or spacing is evaluated through the correlation of dental width and the alveolar bone available. The symmetry between the left and right half in the upper and lower dental arches in all three dimensions is assessed, since there might be asymmetries at the vertical level that concern teeth, groups of teeth or the whole of the dental arch, causing an inclination to the transverse occlusal plane. The orientation of the occlusal plane is assessed on the basis of the curve of Spee in regard to the anteroposterior dimension, and on the basis of the curve of Wilson frontally (Fig. 4). In cases of posterior cross-bite with an increased curve of Wilson, it is very difficult or impossible to achieve proper occlusion with orthodontic, orthopaedic or even surgical maxillary expansion. The solution for such cases is maxillary expansion with multiple section osteotomies. Buccal inclination of posterior lower teeth is often associated with macroglossia or tongue protrusion (Wolford et al., 2004).

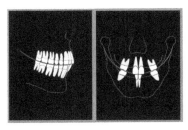

Fig. 4. The curve of Spee and of Wilson

Assessment of the width of the upper and lower dental arches is performed by measuring the inter-canine, inter-premolar and inter-molar distances and comparing them with the recommended normal values, which, however, is purely indicative in nature and changes depending on race and an individual's size. Disorders in the transverse plane affect preoperative orthodontics and determine the surgical treatment necessary. A practical way to reveal width discrepancies, as well as upper and lower arch discrepancies in general, is to mount the casts manually, so that the first molars are in Class I malocclusion.

Casts help us perform Bolton analysis, which is a method that compares the magnitude of the mesio-distal dimension of the upper and lower teeth. It may concern the anterior teeth or the whole set of teeth of the two arches. If there are discrepancies in tooth width, alignment and intercuspation are obstructed. Such disorders are usually caused by small upper lateral incisors or wide lower ones. Along with Bolton analysis, one should take into account the incisors' labiolingual width and their axial inclination. Assessing tooth size discrepancies is very important because this is also a factor determining the goals of presurgical orthodontics and surgical treatment. An even more accurate assessment is possible with a diagnostic wax set up on the casts.

A pair of casts is mounted on an anatomical articulator with facebow record, although a hinge articulator might be suitable for cases that require only mandibular surgery. The need to mount casts during the initial stages of treatment planning is a controversial issue, but may be necessary if maxillary impaction is being planned, so as to define the effect of mandibular autorotation. In cases of significant displacement, it might also be useful to mount casts in central occlusion so as to help treatment planning. In most cases, however, it is sufficient to use manual mounting of casts so as to determine arch intercuspation, avoiding the need of a facebow record (Winchester & Young, 2007).

5.2 Photographs

Photographs are an auxiliary tool for the clinical examination and cephalometry when investigating the aesthetic and functional restoration of the dentition and the face. Initially, two frontal photographs should be taken, one with the lips at rest position and one with the person laughing; then a ¾ photograph of the face and a profile photograph should taken. In cases of asymmetries, it would be useful to take photographs of both profiles. In order to make better use of extra-oral photographs, hair, beard and moustache should be removed from the face. Intra-oral photographs should include anterior teeth and the left and right buccal segments parts in occlusion as well as photographs of the occlusal surfaces of the upper and lower arch using a mirror. Photographs sometimes provide a more objective view than clinical examination, particularly in cases of asymmetry. Photographs should be taken before and after surgery to help the intervention or to serve teaching purposes; rarely, they might also be used for medico-legal purposes.

5.3 Radiographs

In order to plan an orthognathic case, it is necessary to have a panoramic and a lateral cephalometric radiograph. The overview of the panoramic radiograph indicates the presence of pathological conditions, such as impacted teeth that have not erupted, congenitally missing teeth or supernumerary teeth, caries, periodontal disease, apical lesions or cysts as well as the inclination or course of dental roots. The panoramic radiograph provides images of various forms of the mandibular open or closed angle as well as the relative position, morphology and integrity of the condyles (Fig. 5). In cases of condyledamage, the radiograph should be complemented by axial tomography or even three dimensional scans of the temporomandibular joint (3 - dimensional CT scan) (Kapila et al., 2011). Periapical radiographs are useful for a more accurate evaluation of inter-root spaces, when inter-dental osteotomies are to be performed. An occlusal radiography is often useful to clarify regions with a particular pathology, e.g. in order to locate the position of impacted teeth and to determine bone deficits in cleft cases.

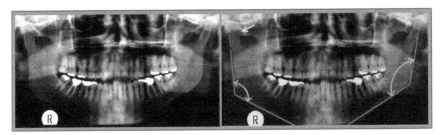

Fig. 5. Panoramic radiograph of a patient with asymmetry

5.3.1 Lateral cephalometric radiograph

Cephalometric analysis performed on the lateral cephalometric radiograph provides details about skeletal structure relationships as well as relationships between skeletal structures and the teeth and facial soft tissues, which cannot be observed in any other way. The catalytic role of such imaging on the complexity of the stomatognathic system and the knowledge of the functional impact of various facial patterns has been included not only in orthodontics but in other fields as well, such as orthognathic surgery.

Although cephalometric analysis is extremely useful to provide information concerning the diagnosis and treatment plan, this is not an absolutely exact scientific method (Baumrind & Frantz, 1971). Furthermore, it should not be considered as a primary diagnostic tool; it should be considered that the treatment aims are a proportional and harmonious facial structure, without necessarily aspiring at ideal cephalometric measurements. When there are significant discrepancies between clinical evaluation and cephalometric analysis data, the clinical assessment is much more significant in preparing the treatment plan (Chaconas & Fragiskos, 1991). Today there is a wide range of cephalometric radiograph analysis methods, which are either linear-descriptive or structural ones (Muller, 1962). Cephalometric radiograph analysis methods are usually based on measurements, which are compared to corresponding ones within normal range; this, however, presents inherent difficulties (Ricketts, 1975; Sassouni 1971), due to racial or ethnic differences, age and gender differences, possible differences in radiographic techniques (orientation in regard to the horizontal Frankfurt plane or in accordance to the natural head position) or differences that concern the criteria for selecting the 'normal' sample, such as occlusal features and skeletal background, at any given time (Miethke, 1995). In essence, though, what is important is whether there is harmony or discrepancy between the functional structures of the craniofacial complex in the same individual rather than the agreement of cephalometric data of the individual under study when compared to the normal sample range, as this was defined by the researcher at any given time (McNamara & Brudon 1993; Sassouni, 1971). Linear and descriptive analysis in lateral cephalometric radiographs is based on the study of jaw relationships with the cranial base and each other, the relationships of teeth with each other and their corresponding bone bases and the relationships of soft tissues in the profile view of the face. Measurements performed concern the maxilla, the mandible, the teeth and soft tissues.

5.3.1.1 Maxillary measurements (Fig. 6)

1. The S-N-A Angle: this provides an indication about the anteroposterior position of the maxillary base in relation to the anterior cranial base. Its normal value is 82°±2 for men and 81°±2 for women. A high value indicates a protruding maxilla, while a low one a retrusive maxilla. 2. The angle formed by the Frankfurt plane and the line defined by the nasion and point A. This is called maxillary depth and its mean value is 90°±3. This angle indicates the anteroposterior position of the maxilla in relation to the horizontal plane. Skeletal Class II type caused by the maxilla presents values over 90°, while, Class III types present lower values. This angle also presents lower values in cases of palatal clefts. 3. The distance of point A from the McNamara line (drawn through point N perpendicularly to the horizontal Frankfurt plane): this indicates the position of the maxilla in relation to the anterior part of the skull and, normally, point A lies near this line. Values above +3 mm indicate maxillary protrusion, while values under –3 mm indicate maxillary retrusion. Anteroposterior maxillary assessment should also take into account that the position of point A is affected by potential alveolar protrusion and by any pronounced inclination of the upper incisors. 4. The N-CF-A Angle (CF is the intersection point of the Frankfurt plane with the PTV plane). This is called maxillary height and its mean value is 56°±3. It indicates the vertical position of the maxilla in the face. In cases of skeletal open bite caused by the maxilla, the values of this angle are low, which indicates a short upper face.

5.3.1.2 Measurements concerning the mandible (Fig. 6)

1. The S-N-B Angle. This indicates the anteroposterior position of the mandible in relation to the anterior base of the skull. Its normal value is 80°±2 for men and 78°±2 for women. A high value indicates a protruding mandible, while a low value a retrusive one. It should be taken into account that the values of the S-N-A and S-N-B angles are influenced by the inclination and lenght of the anterior cranial base S-N. 2. The facial angle, formed by the Frankfurt plane and the facial plane N-Pg. Its mean value is 90°±3. This angle assesses the anteroposterior position of the mandible and determines whether a skeletal Class II or III is caused by the mandible. 3. The distance of point Pg from the vertical line going through point N. This indicates the anteroposterior position of the mandible in relation to the base of the skull. Normally, its values range from -4 mm to 0 mm for individuals of medium facial size (McNamara, 1984). Among adults, point Pg usually lies 2 mm behind this line. Values under –5 mm indicate a retrusive mandible, while values above +3 mm indicate a protrusive maxilla (Stroud, 1997). 4. The angle formed by the mandibular plane (Go-Me) and the Frankfurt plane. This is the FMA Angle of Tweed. Its mean value is 25°±4. This angle provides an indication as to the vertical height of the mandibular ramus and the posterior facial height. This measurement indicates the vertical type of the face. An open angle indicates a long face and, in cases of skeletal anterior open bite, that it is caused by the mandible. On the contrary, a closed angle indicates a short type of face and in cases of skeletal deep bite this is caused by the mandible. A high value indicates a long and narrow face with narrow dental arches. On the contrary, patients with a small angle tend to have a relatively high posterior facial height and increased activity of the masticatory muscles. Furthermore, they have a tendency for an overbite and muscular spasm particularly of the

temporalis and the medial pterygoid muscle, predisposing for TMJ problems (Chaconas & Gonidis, 1986).

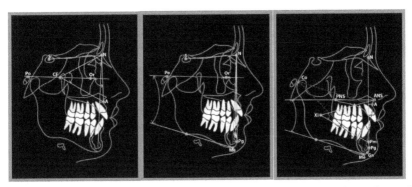

Fig. 6. Cephalometric measurements concerning maxilla, mandible and their relationship

5.3.1.3 Measurements concerning the relationship between maxilla and mandible (Fig.6)

1. The convexity of the face, which is the distance of point A from the facial plane N-Pg. Its mean value among adults is 1.7 mm±2. If point A lies in front of the N-Pg line, then the profile is convex and it is a skeletal Class II case, either because the chin is retrusive or because the maxilla is protruding or because there is a combination of the two. On the contrary, if point A lies behind the N-Pg line, then the profile is concave and the case is one of skeletal Class III, either because the chin is protruding or because the maxilla is retrusive or because the two conditions co-exist. The highest acceptable convexity among adults is 4 mm (Langlande, 1981). 2. The ANS-Xi-Pm angle indicates the lower facial height. Its mean value among adults is 47°±4. If this angle value is higher, it indicates the presence of open bite, while a lower value indicates the presence of deep bite. 3. The angle formed by the maxillary plane (ANS-PNS) and the mandibular plane (Go-Me). Its mean value is 27°±4. This angle is important because it indicates the posterior facial height and reflects the surgically significant pterygo-masticatory muscle and ligament height. For example, a patient with a high value for this angle, e.g. exceeding 35°, tends to have a relatively short posterior facial height and, therefore, an equally short posterior height of the muscles and ligaments involved. Any attempts to stretch this posterior connective tissue by rotating the anterior mandibular body upwards, in an anti-clockwise direction, around a fulcrum formed by the posterior molar occlusion is condemned to fail and lead to early surgical relapse (Hunt, 2008a). It should be noted here that the position of the mandible is not only affected by its size and its position due to the inclination of the cranial base, but also by the vertical dimension. For example, if the vertical dimension is excessive, the mandible might appear to be insufficient in relation to the maxilla. Therefore, it would be relatively retrusive, but only due to the vertical dimenstion. The opposite would be true in vertical deficits. If the vertical dimension is not normal, additional measurements often help clarify the analysis (Stroud LP. (1997), such as those recommended in McNamara's method. McNamara's method (McNamara, 1984) attempts to individualise patients, given that there is indeed a stable linear relationship between the relative length of the maxilla (distance between Condyle Co, i.e. the most superior lateral point of the mandibular condyle, and point A) and the relative length of the mandible (distance between the Condylium Co from the anatomical Gn). For

every relative length of the maxilla of a specific individual, there is one relative length of the mandible within a given width. This relationship also takes into account the vertical dimension, as this is defined by the anterior lower facial height (ANS-Me) (Fig. 6). In other words, what is characteristic about the McNamara method is the presence of the triangle formed by the maxilla, the mandible and the anterior lower facial height and their interrelationship as shown in the tables of composite values resulting from the combination of the three cephalometric samples (Table 1). So, the "originality" of this method lies in the fact that it directly correlates maxillary and mandibular lengths with lower facial height, regardless of the gender or the age of an individual. This leads to a useful combination of measurements with the substantial advantage of using it for diagnostic and therapeutic purposes in cases of skeletal problems, particularly when a combination of orthodontic treatment and orthognathic surgery is required (Sinclair & Proffit, 1991).

5.3.1.4 Measurements concerning dental relations (Fig. 7)

1. The angle formed by the lognitudinal axis of the upper incisor and the palatal plane (1/ANS-PNS). Its mean value is 109°±5. In cases of Class III dentoalveolar disorder, this angle often presents increased values, since the incisors have an increased labial inclination in order to compensate for or alleviate the malocclusion present. 2. The angle formed by the lognitudinal axis of the upper incisor and the anterior cranial base (1/S-N). Its mean value is 103°±2. This angle becomes particularly significant in cases when the palatal plane is to surgically change inclination, as in some open bite cases. In these cases, its coassessment with Angle 1/ANS-PNS indicates to the orthodontist the necessary preoperative movement of upper incisors. 3. The distance of the labial surface of the upper incisor from a vertical line going through point A and drawn so as to be parallel to the vertical line going through the nasion. This measurement determines the anteroposterior position of the upper incisor in relation to the mandible. Its mean value is 4-6 mm. Upper incisor positions more posterior than 1 mm to this line are considered to be lingual positions, while upper incisors situated more than 7 mm anterior to this line are prominent incisors. 4. The angle formed by the lognitudinal axis of the lower incisor and the mandibular base plane (ī /Go-Me). Its mean value is 90°±5. This angle indicates the anatomical position of the lower incisor in relation to the base of the mandible. A reduced value of this angle is almost always encountered in Class III malocclusion cases, as a compensatory factor. However, in cases of Class II malocclusion, this angle is increased (Guariglia & Ronchi, 2005). 5. The angle formed by the lognitudinal axis of the lower incisor and the dentoalveolar plane A-Pg (ī /A-Pg). Its mean value is 22°±4. This angle indicates the inclination of the lower incisor in relation to the

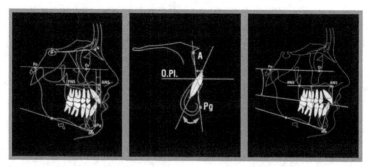

Fig. 7. Cephalometric measurements concerning dental relationships

dentoalveolar plane A-Pg and it adapts to the facial skeletal type; it is increased in short facial types and decreased in long types. 6. The distance of the lower incisal edge from the dentoalveolar plane A-Pg ($\bar{\imath}$ →A-Pg). Its mean value is 2.4 mm±2 and it indicates the projection of the lower incisor. Incisors lying more than 5 mm in front of the line are protruding, while incisors behind the line are retrusive. 7. The distance of the lower incisal edge from the occlusal plane. Its mean value is 1.25 mm±2 and it indicates overeruption of the lower incisor; it shows whether the abnormal deep bite is due to theintrusion orextrusion of the lower or upper incisor (Ricketts, 1982). 8. The distance of the upper incisal edge from the palatal plane ($\underline{1}$ →ANS-PNS). Its mean value is 33 mm±3 and it indicates the anterior dentoalveolar height. 9. The distance of the lower incisal edge from the mandibular plane ($\bar{\imath}$ →Go-Me). Its mean value is 44 mm±2 for men and 40 mm±2 for women. It indicates the lower anterior dentoalveolar height. It should be noted that these measurements of the anterior upper and lower dentoalveolar height reflect aspects of the lower height of the face. In other words, if the anterior lower height of the face is increased, then the upper and lower anterior dentoalveolar height will also be increased, with the exception of some open bite cases. (Hunt, 2008a). 10. The distance of the tip of the medial cusp of the lower first molar from the mandibular plane ($\bar{6}$ →Go-Me). Its mean value is 38 mm±3 and it indicates the posterior lower dentoalveolar height. 11. The distance of the tip of the medial cusp of the upper first molar from the palatal plane ($\underline{6}$ →ANS-PNS). Its mean value is 28 mm±3 and it indicates the posterior upper dentoalveolar height. Low values of the upper and lower posterior dentoalveolar height might indicate ankylosis or eruption failure. On the contrary, high values indicate supraeruption and are blamed for skeletal anterior open bite (Langlande, 1986). 12. The angle formed by the occlusal plane and the horizontal Frankfurt plane. The occlusal plane is defined by points corresponding to the middle of the overlapping of the cusps of premolars and molars. Mean angle value is 8°±4 and it indicates the inclination of the occlusal plane. This plane is very important from a functional point of view, in relation to mandibular movement. Along with the anterior and posterior decisive factors for occlusion, it determines how teeth get disengaged (Stroud, 1997). The occlusal plane has a significant impact on function and aesthetics, particularly in cases of bimaxillary osteotomy (Wolford, 2007).

5.3.1.5 Measurements concerning facial soft tissues (Fig. 8)

1. The ratio of the middle third to the lower third of facial soft tissues is 1:1. The middle third is the distance determined by points Gs (the most anterior part of the forehead corresponding to the glabella) and Sn (the most posterior point of the nasal base, where it joins the upper lip). The lower third is the distance defined by points Sn and Mes (the lowest point of chin soft tissues). In most orthognathic surgery patients, abnormalities are located in the lower third of the face, which is increased in relation to the middle third, either due to vertical excess of the posterior maxillary region or due to increased anterior vertical height of the mandible. In cases of reduced lower third of the face, the cause expected is either vertical maxillary hypoplasia or reduction of the anterior vertical height of the mandible or forward rotation of the mandible (Reyneke, 2003). 2. The length and eminence of the nose is the projection of the Sn - Pn distance on a straight line parallel to the horizontal Frankfurt plane and going through point Sn. Its mean value is 18±2 mm. Aesthetically it is more acceptable for women to have less eminent noses than men (Lines et al., 1978). When planning maxillary osteotomy, the impact it might have on the nose should be taken into account. 3. The distance of the subnasal point Sn from point Sts (the lowest point of the

upper lip) is the upper lip height. Its normal value is 22±2 mm in men and 20±2 mm in women. If measurements indicate values below normal ones, then the upper lip is short. The upper lip height is a decisive factor for the vertical dimensions of the lower third of the face, because it represents one third of this distance and because it is not easy for the upper lip height to change. This measurement is the basis that can determine the vertical height of the lower two thirds of the lower third of the face.

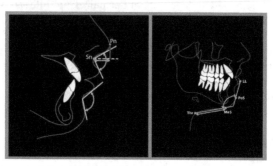

Fig. 8. Measurements concerning facial soft tissues

4. The distance of point Sts from the upper incisal edge, when the lips are at rest. Its normal value is 2.5 ± 1.5 mm (Arnett & Bergman, 1993; Fish & Epker, 1980; Miethke, 1995; Proffit, 1993). This measurement is affected by the upper lip height, the height of the maxilla, the height of the upper incisal crown, the thickness of the lips and the inclination and anteroposterior position of the upper incisors. This assessement is particularly important when determining the vertical dimensions of the face, particularly when there are vertical maxillary dysplasia (Wolford, 2007). Lack of upper incisor exposure might indicate vertical maxillary hypoplasia, while exposure exceeding 4 mm may indicate vertical maxillary excess, if the the upper lip height is normal (Reyneke, 2003). 5. The nasolabial angle, formed by a tangent on the columella which goes through the subnasal point Sn and a straight line connecting point Sn with the most anterior point of the upper lip (UL). An angle of 85°-105° is considered normal and this value varies depending on race (Burstone, 1967; Lines et al., 1978). The angle is usually acute in Class III cases, while Class II patients present a more obtuse nasolabial angle. A straight line going through point Sn and parallel to the horizontal plane separates the nasolabial angle into a superior and an inferior part. The upper/lower nasolabial angle ratio is of particular importance and should be one to four (Fig. 8). Ratios above 25% indicate an eminent upper lip or an upward tipping nose. On the contrary, lower ratios may indicate a retrusive upper lip or reduced eminence of the nose tip (Stella & Epker, 1990). It should be taken into account that when the maxilla is surgically shifted upward and backward, this causes loss of upper lip support, an increased nasolabial angle and flattening of the nose, which results in bad aesthetics due to a premature aging effect. 6. The mentolabial angle, formed by the straight line that goes through the most posterior point of the mentolabial sulcus (Sm) and it is tangent to the lower lip and the chin tangent that also goes through point Sm. Its mean value is 130°±10, with lower values preferable for men than for women. This angle is usually acute in Class II cases with anteroposterior mandibular hypoplasia, due to the pressure exercised by the upper incisors on the lower lip or in cases of macrogenia. The angle is flattened in microgenia cases or due to lower lip tension in Class III malocclusion cases. When planning genioplastic osteotomy, what should

be considered is not only the anteroposterior position of the chin but also the menton shape and the mentolabial sulcus. 7. The mentocervical angle, formed by the straight line going through the most posterior point of the menton (PoS) and the most anterior point of the lower lip (LL) and a straight line going through the lowest point of the menton (MeS) and the neck-throat joint point (Thr). The mean value of this angle is 110°±8. It is more acute in skeletal Class III cases and less acute in skeletal Class II cases, in which mandibular disorders are involved. 8. The throat length is the distance between the neck-throat joint point (Thr) and the lowest point of the menton (MeS). Its mean value is 40±5 mm. The throat length is increased in cases of mandibular macrognathia and it is shorter in cases of mandibular micrognathia. This measurement is useful to ensure differential diagnosis between anteroposterior mandibular excess and maxillary hypoplasia. The menton-throat angle and the throat length are of particular importance when planning surgical anteroposterior shift of the mandible, genioplastic osteotomy (protrusive or reductive) or submental liposuction. Thus, in individuals with a short throat length and mandibular protrusion, backward surgical shift of the mandible would be particularly unaesthetic (Proffit, 1991). To ensure proper assessment of these measurements, radiographs should be taken in the natural head position. 9. The eminence of the upper and lower lips and the chin are assessed on the basis of distances of points UL, LL and PoS from a straight line that goes through point Sn and is perpendicular to the Frankfurt plane. Mean values of these distances are as follows: 2±2 mm for the upper lip, 0±2 mm for the lower lip and -3.5±2 mm for the chin (Bass, 1991: Fish & Epker, 1980; Wolford, 1990). The eminence of the lips, according to Ricketts are the distances of points UL and LL from the aesthetic plane PoS-Pn. Normally, the lips lie behind the aesthetic plane: the upper lip at 4 mm and the lower lip at 2 mm. These measurements indicate the balance or lack of balance of the soft tissue between the lips and the nose - chin profile (Ricketts et al., 1982).

5.3.1.6 Cephalometric prediction of surgical orthodontic treatment

Cephalometric prediction of the surgical orthodontic treatment outcome allows the direct visualization of both dental and skeletal movement and projects the probable post-surgical patient profile. It can be of assistance to both orthodontists and maxillofacial surgeon in planning the treatment and to patients in comprehending postoperative changes and, mainly, the change in the appearance of their faces. Various manual cephalometric methods have been proposed (Fish & Epker 1980; McNeil et al., 1972; Proffit, 1991; Wolford et al., 1985; Worms, 1976). Manual cephalometric techniques are implemented either using the overlay method or templates. The overlay method by Proffit (Proffit, 1991) is the simplest prediction method for mandibular osteotomies; it is restricted to surgeries that do not affect the vertical position of the maxilla and is not time consuming. These are its stages, in brief (Fig. 9) : a) drawing the initial cephalometric tracing (CT) and the surgical reference line; b) a second acetate paper is placed over the initial tracing, so called the overlay tracing; Drawing on the overlay tracing the skeletal structures that are not going to change during surgery, including the surgical reference line; c) Movement of the CT mandible backward, on the overlay so as to achieve the desirable overjet and overbite and the proper intercuspation of posterior teeth. Drawing on the overlay the lower teeth and the part of the mandible in front of the surgical line; d) Superimposition on the cranial base and measurement of the backward movement of the lower incisor and skeletal chin movement; calculation of the predicted position of the lower lip and soft chin, using data regarding ratios of soft tissue changes relative to respective skeletal movements (the response of the lower lip represents 60% of skeletal changes, while the chin response is absolute, i.e. 1:1)

(Jensen et al., 1992). Measurement of the distance between the surgical reference lines to determine the surgical movement in millimetres; e) Superimposition at the mandible and drawing the lower lip outline and the chin; f) Superimposition at the cranial base; drawing the predicted soft tissue profile. The template method is implemented in all types of osteotomy and it is very useful in repositioning of the chin and almost necessary when the maxilla is plan to be moved on the vertical plane. However, the implementation of this method is time-consuming. In cases of one or two pieces osteotomies, the entire maxilla outline is drawn while in three-piece osteotomies an outline of the anterior and posterior maxillary pieces and the mandibular outline are drawn. The mandible rotates around the condyle (Proffit & Sarver, 2003).

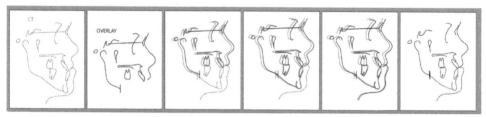

Fig. 9. The stages of Proffit's overlay method

Cephalometric prediction using a computer presupposes digital tracing of the cephalometric radiograph; it can be performed either by using software programmes alone or a combination of software and video images (Athanasiou & Kragskov, 1995). The operator shifts the cursor to various points, depending on the type of surgery, until the desirable aesthetic outcome is achieved. Then the predicted postoperative profile is printed and surgical movements can be calculated on it. This way, it is possible to save and analyse graphic data, to diagnose and plan the orthognathic cases as well as to predict the patient's postoperative profile. Computerized cephalometric prediction combined with video images is performed through automatic superimposition of the cephalogram on the patient's profile by the software programme, which is visible on the video monitor. All movements are of actual size. Today three-dimensional prediction methods are available. Computer prediction facilitates physician-patient communication, but there are certain inaccuracies involving mainly the lip area and the chin region (Eales et al., 1994; Kaipatur & Flores-Mir, 2009; Kolokitha et al., 1996; Kolokitha, 2007).

5.3.2 Anteroposterior cephalometric radiography

Anteroposterior analysis based on cephalometric radiographs is mainly useful for studying transverse asymmetries of the craniofacial complex. This analysis provides information about the width and inclination of the dental arches in relation to their osseous bases at the transverse plane. The analysis also provides an opportunity to assess the width of transverse maxillomandiubular relations and the vertical dimensions of corresponding skeletal parts or points of the dentition of the two facial halves and the nasal cavity, while analysing any asymmertries at the transverse or vertical planes. The study of facial symmetry is not always a mathematical measurement, according to certain authors. The symmetry can also be 'roughly' assessed, i.e. just by looking at the face. Vion considers it easier to assess asymmetry by placing the tracing on millimetre graph paper (Vion, 1976). Ricketts recommends the use of measurements, the most important of which for orthognathic surgery candidates are the following (Ricketts, 1982) (Fig. 10): 1. The distance between the maxilla (zygomatic process) and the frontal facial plane (JR →ZR) and (JL →ZL). Its mean value for adults is 15±1.5 mm and it indicates the left and right width of the maxilla and the mandible. It determines whether posterior cross-bite is skeletal. High values indicate skeletal lingual cross-bite, while low values indicate skeletal buccal cross-bite. 2. The angle formed by the maxillary midline (ANS – middle of ZR – ZL) and the mandibular midline (ANS - Me). Its mean value is 0°±2. In cases of asymmetry, this angle determines whether it is caused by dental or skeletal causes or by functional shift of the mandible. When the two midlines coincide there is symmetry and they both go through the incisal contact points. 3. The difference between the height of the occlusal plane at the left and right molars, measured in relation to the ZR – ZL line. Its mean value is 0±2 mm. Deviation from the mean value indicates asymmetry accompanied by structural abnormality of the maxilla or the mandible or both jaws. True skeletal asymmetry accompanied by an inclined occlusal plane is usually a warning sign for TMJ dysfunction. 4. The difference between the right and left angles, formed by points ZR-GA-AZ on the right and ZL-AG-ZA on the left. Its mean value is 0°±2. It indicates the position of the mandible and helps explain the nature of the asymmetry. Where the difference exceeds 4° it should be examined whether the asymmetry is of a structural or functional aetiology. These angles are significantly affected by a head turn on the headrest. Langlande also recommends the use of the distance between point DC (top of the condyle head) and the corresponding anti-gonion point AG, as well as the distance between point Me and the corresponding anti-gonion point so as to assess asymmetry (Fig. 10). These measurements make it possible to judge whether the asymmetry is due to the ramus or the body of the mandible (Langlande, 1981).

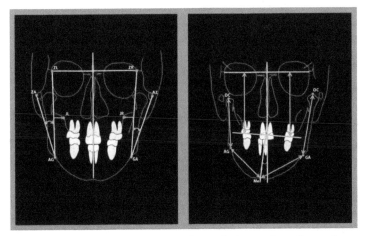

Fig. 10. Measurements concerning anteroposterior cephalometric radiographs

6. Preoperative orthodontics

The goals of preoperative orthodontic treatment are to allow for maximum surgical correction of the abnormality, to facilitate potential sectional surgical procedures and to provide the possibility for creating an ideal, stable occlusion (Tompach et al., 1995). The major part of orthodontic treatment takes place before surgery and might last one and a half to two years (Slavnic & Marcusson, 2010; Diaz et al., 2010). However, there are those who prefer to leave the major part of orthodontic treatment for after the surgery. Extensive preoperative treatment and limited postoperative treatment is usually better tolerated by the patient and provides smoother cooperation (Lee, 1994). The goals of preoperative orthodontic treatment are achieved with the alignment and flattening of the arches, the exacerbation of dental relations by removing all dentoalveolar compensation for the skeletal abnormality and with arch coordination.

6.1 Arch alignment

The first goal of preoperative orthodontics is to align the dental arches or their parts so that they might be compatible with each other. Correcting crowding and rotations, management of impacted teeth and arch length discrepancies is mainly a concern of preoperative orthodontics, because it facilitates arch intercuspation; otherwise, the surgical result would be restricted. If arch length is to be reduced, and the incisors need to be shifted backwards, then extractions are performed, as, for example, in Class III cases, when the upper incisors need to be moved backward or in Class II cases, when the lower incisors have to be moved backward to achieve exacerbation (Proffit & White, 1991) (Fig. 11). When sectional surgery is being planned, the deviation of dental roots close to the osteotomies starts with the initial wire and it is monitored through periapical radiographs. The modern preconstructed brackets of fixed devices and straight Ni-Ti wires have significantly simplified modern orthodontics. Selecting the slot size is a matter of personal preference, although the 0.022 inch system can better immobilise intraoperatively with rigid 19 X 25 wires. Ceramic brackets are pleasant, because they provide aesthetic solutions; however, their disadvantage is that they break easily during surgical manipulations. Most preconstructed bracket systems have been designed to tip the roots of canines distally and, thus, create sufficient space between them and the roots of lateral incisors.

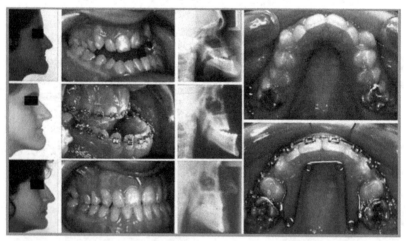

Fig. 11. A Class III case, with preoperative extractions of the first upper premolars to manage crowding and to move the upper incisors in order to achieve exacerbation of the negative overjet, which was completed with labial tipping of the lower incisors

This space is useful in cases where interdental osteotomies are to take place in the maxilla. When osteotomy incisions are performed distally to the canines, the use of brackets on the contralateral canines warrants that the integrated distal tipping of the brackets keeps the apices anteriorly and outside surgical incisions (Hunt, 2008b).

6.2 Arch flattening

The planning of dental arch flattening is particularly important. The general principle is that extrusion is easier postoperatively, while intrusion needs to be completed preoperatively or intra-operatively. Dental flattening and alignment are ususally a common one-step process in conventional orthodontics. This is not the case for all surgical cases. When the mandible is surgically moved forward or backward, the position of the lower incisor is what determines the lower facial height. In surgical correction of Class II, when the lower facial height is reduced, it is preferable not to correct the curve of Spee in the lower dental arch, either through orthodontics or surgically. Surgical protrusion of the mandible creates lateral open bite and a tripod-like occlusal relation; only the last molars and incisors are in an occlusal relationship. Besides, the lower facial height increases as the chin moves downward. Before the operation, the teeth are aligned and the anteroposterior relationship of the incisors has been determined. However, the curve of Spee remains in all wire arches, including the final stabilising wire (Proffit & Fields, 2007). The lateral open bite is treated with extrusion of the teeth involved, using vertical elastic forces during postoperative orthodontics. Numerous clinicians think that 2mm of extrusion in every arch is the maximum that may be achieved and remain stable without relapse (Hunt, 2008b). If the intentional lateral open bite that remains after surgery is deemed to be too much, then the curve of Spee will have to be reduced preoperatively, with the inevitable limitation that the increment of the lower anterior facial height will be limited postoperatively.

If the incisors are intruded preoperatively in a patient with deep bite, the operation tends to move the mandible upwards at the chin and downwards in the menton region, due to pivot effect. This increase of the posterior facial height will stretch the masticatory muscles (muscular stretching) and this is why it is unstable. However, when the incisors are not intruded preoperatively, the operation will move the chin downwards and the mandibular angle upwards, thus causing clockwise rotation of the mandible, which, generally speaking, is more stable in relation to the anti-clockwise mandibular rotation (Lake et al., 1981). (Fig. 12). On the contrary, when the lower facial height is increased, the pronounced curve of Spee has to be flattened preoperatively by intrution of the anterior part or surgically flattened with base osteotomy following sectional orthodontic flattening. Often a combined operation involving the maxilla is necessary to avoid the downward movement of the menton angle and further increase of the facial height, which is undesirable. If intrusion is necessary, the technique of sectional arches is indicated for preoperative orthodontics using mild forces in the order of 10 - 20 g per tooth, so that root resorption may be avoided, particularly if the teeth are fine. If this approach leads to lack of dental position control, it is preferable to have a continuous arch from molar to molar, with an anterior step for the incisors and canines. Continuous straight arches may achieve flattening, but probably with undesirable incisor tipping, which can be managed with extractions that allow the posterior movement of incisors. Surgical flattening is rarely indicated for the lower dental arch (Hunt, 2008b; Levander & Malmgren, 1988). When surgically correcting open bite, in cases of increased lower facial height, it is preferable not to correct the curve of Spee preoperatively in the upper dental arch, since multiple section osteotomies are indicated in such cases. During preoperative orthodontics, the aim is to exacerbate open bite with extrusion of posterior teeth and intrusion of anterior ones. During the operation, the final flattening of sections takes place, which allows the forward rotation of the mandible. If a one piece Le Fort I osteotomy is decided, with greater intrusion of the posterior part of the maxilla, preoperative orthodontic flattening is required, but anterior teeth extrusion should be avoided before the operation, because even mild orthodontic relapse may cause postoperative opening of the bite (Proffit & Fields, 2007). The importance of orthodontic movements of sectional flattening, which are usually unstable, is that it allows an attempt to minimise postoperative relapse. Following the removal of fixed orthodontic devices, the intruded incisors tend to infraocclude again and the extruded molars and premolars tend to intrude once again, thus compensating for the trend of the open bite to recur as a result of surgical relapse or undesirable growth rotation. (Houston, 1988; Lake et al., 1981). Sectional flattening is achieved if a step is made preoperatively to the upper wire arch at the occlusal plane or two lateral and one labial sectional arches are inserted. Other orthodontic devices that may be used are upper wire arches with increased curve of Spee, lower wire arches with inversed curve of Spee, inter-arch elastics to extrude posterior teeth, neck-traction headgear on the upper molars, J-pull headgear on the upper incisors or mini screws in order to intrude them (Winchester & Young, 2007).

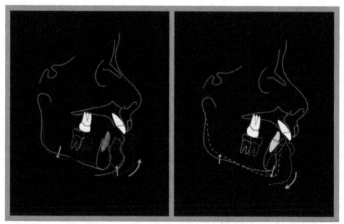

Fig. 12. Schematic representation of a Class II case surgical correction, where there is reduced lower facial height and the curve of Spee is pronounced. The red colour indicates chin and menton movements if the incisors are intruded (A) preoperatively and the green colour indicates what happens if they are not (B).

6.3 Exacerbation
In serious skeletal discrepancies, the teeth try to maintain some contact, under the effect of external and internal forces, so as to compensate for the skeletal problem. Although this compensation improves occlusal relationships and the patient's appearance, it restricts the extent of surgical correction. In skeletal Class III cases, the upper incisors are often labially inclined, while the lower ones are lingually inclined. On the contrary, in cases of skeletal Class II the upper incisors are often upright and the lower labially inclined. A consequence of these compensatory changes is that the overjet is virtual in regard to the actual magnitude of the skeletal discrepancy. Preoperative orthodontics aims at exacerbating dental

relationships, by removing the camouflage effect and placing the incisors in normal inclination for the skeletal bases, if this is feasible (Jacobs & Sinclair, 1983). (Fig. 20, 21) Removing compensation exacerbates the malocclusion preoperatively, but reveals the true magnitude of the skeletal problem, thus allowing optimal surgical correction without limitations or occlusal interference. So, if dental compensation from the incisors in Class II, type 1 cases is removed, twice as much forward movement of the mandible is possible, as opposed to what would have achieved if the compensation had not been removed. Similarly, in Class III cases, the mandibular backward movement allowed is five times as much when compensation is removed. (Fig. 13) (Worms et al., 1976). In Class II, type 1 cases, extractions of the first lower premolars may be performed to achieve exacerbation (Fig. 13) and Class III inter-gnathic elastic forces may be used. In Class III cases, there is often a small maxilla with crowding and the upper first premolars might have to be extracted along with the expansion, so as to achieve exacerbation. Furthermore, in Class III cases, when the goal is anteroposterior exacerbation, Class II inter-gnathic elastic forces may be used (Jacobs & Sinclair, 1983). The use of Roth's brackets on incisors with increased crown torque might be an advantage in Class II cases, but undesirable in surgical Class III cases (Winchester & Young, 2007). The exacerbation extent of the incisors is affected by postoperative skeletal stability; this means that full and extensive exacerbation might not always be the goal for a sound surgical outcome. In a Class III case, the exacerbation of the incisors might lead to such great discrepancy, that two-jaw osteotomy might be required for correction and a stable postoperative outcome; on the contrary, limited compensation might only need mandibular surgery. Furthermore, the extent of the exacerbation is restricted in cases of insufficient alveolar bone, when the roots of the incisors are fine or partly resorbed or if there are teeth with poor prognosis. When there is a very narrow attached gum zone or thin periodontium in the lower anterior region, it might be advisable to place a free gum graft before labial dental movement, so as to avoid resorption of the labial alveolar process and denuding of the roots (Boyd, 1978). In the case of maxillary depression at different levels, full exacerbation of the upper incisors is not necessary. The posterior region of the maxilla is depressed more than its anterior part. The consequence of such surgery is that the incisors are palatally inclined. So, when orthodontics is performed in this case, preoperative preparation migth intentionally leave the upper incisors with a slight labial inclination (Hunt N, 2008b).

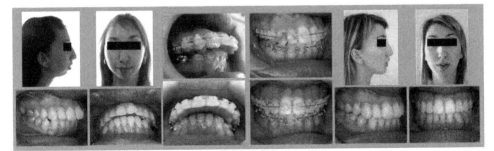

Fig. 13. A Class II case, where the lower anterior teeth, after extractions of the first lower premolars, were moved backwards to achieve exacerbation and allow forward surgical movement of the mandible. During postoperative treatment, Class II elastic forces were used to support sagittal correction.

6.4 Intercuspation of the two arches

One of the goals of preoperative orthodontics is to achieve harmonisation of dental arches at all levels during surgery. Controlling dental arch harmonisation is initially achieved by the use of snap models (mounting the casts manually in occlusion) before surgery. Anteroposterior changes in skeletal relationships sometimes require modification in the transverse width of the arches, and expansion of the upper dental arch, in particular, so as to achieve harmonisation of intermolar and intercanine width. The way to achieve expansion depends on its magnitude and the initial bucco-lingual inclination of upper posterior teeth. Usually, this occurs spontaneously with the use of coordinated upper and lower continuous wire arches and the quad-helix device, which are useful for progressive expansion (Proffit & White, 2003). The quad helix device might result in a deviating movement, but it has the advantage of allowing differential expansion in the right and left buccal sections. Rapid maxillary expansion is not recommended for adults, dut to potential risk for the roots and the periodontium, although surgically assisted rapid maxillary expansion may be performed (Barber & Sims, 1981).

Transverse problems are often overlooked because posterior dental compensation is less apparent than sagittal skeletal discrepancies of the incisors. However, these become apparent during simulated cast surgery. In surgery simulation of a serious skeletal Class II case, by moving the initial casts manually, a bilateral cross-bite occlusion appears, which was not apparent before, because the lower arch has moved to a narrower region of the upper arch. On the contrary, a posterior cross-bite in Class III may not need preoperative management, because it might well be resolved automatically with the posterior surgical mandibular movement, as the lower arch moves to a wider part of the upper arch or as the upper arch moves to a narrower part of the lower arch in cases of surgical maxillary protrusion. Furthermore, in Class III cases with narrow upper arches, the palatal cusps of the molars often interfere with the postoperative position planned, due to insufficient control of the torque. The use of Roth's molar rings with increased torque helps prevent this problem. Thick, rigid, rectangular wire arches are necessary to control torque and maintain the expansion achieved (Winchester & Young, 2007). The transverse problem needs to be diagnosed from the start. It is also essential to note if it is of dental or skeletal aetiology and if correction is to be achieved through orthodontics, sectional surgery or surgically assisted palatal expansion. Orthodontic expansion should not be attempted preoperatively in patients who are going to undergo surgical expansion. Finally, the only way to check if arch compatibility has been achieved in surgical patients is to mount the study casts on the articulator (Sabri, 2006).

Before the end of the preoperative phase, upper and lower rigid rectangular wires need to be passively in position for eight weeks before surgery. Some type of hooks or brackets with thick attachments should be placed on the wires Kobayashi so as to facilitate immobilisation during surgery. Preoperative orthodontics should have been completed in twelve months and the case needs to be planned in such a way for postoperative treatment, that the final correction may be achieved within six months.

7. Postoperative orthodontics

The aim of postoperative orthodontics is to bring the teeth to their final positions and secure balanced occlusion; finally retention planning should be achieved. This phase of the treatment starts two to four weeks later, after a satisfactory range of mandibular movement has been achieved and there is good bone healing. At first the occlusal splint is removed as well as the rigid stabilising wires, which are replaced by continuous working wires. This replacement is quite significant, particularly when there are occlusal surfaces only in two or three teeth after the splint is removed, which means that proprioceptive stimuli make the patient try to find a new position with more contact points. This, however, is not desirable because it might complicate the completion of treatment and the healing of recent osteotomies. This problem is avoided if teeth are allowed to freely come to full contact immediately after splint removal. This is better achieved with light, round wires combined with light, box elastics (Sabri, 2006). Postoperative correction of tripod occlusion with a pronounced curve of Spee and lateral open bite usually includes a combination of elastic wire arches with vertical intergnathic elastics and may last slightly longer than usual. When the upper dental arch is flat, a stable upper rectangular arch is maintained, while an elastic arch, for example a braided steel wire, may be placed on the lower arch. When both arches need extrusion, the rectangular arches may be cut and elastics can be applied between the upper and lower sections (Hunt, 2008b). The elastics are not necessarily vertical, but can have an anterior or posterior contributing force to support sagittal correction. For mandibular protrusion Class II elastics should be used (Fig. 13), whereas mandibular retrusion needs Class III elastics. The orthodontist needs to see the patient every two to three weeks at this stage, to continue the controlled guidance towards final occlusion relationships through the elastics and to avoid displacement or deviations of the mandible. Usually patients wear the elastics continously, even when eating, for the first four weeks, continuously but not at meal times for the next four weeks and only at night for another four weeks (Proffit & Fields, 2007). In cases with a predisposition for open bite, postoperative use of elastics in the buccal sections needs to last the shortest possible time, so as to avoid opening the bite. The use of elastics is terminated after stable occlusion has been achieved. In cases when multiple section osteotomies have been performed and the canine brackets had been preoperatively reversed, it is necessary for them to be reattached, by placing them in the proper position so as to create the right deviation of their longitudinal axes. If palatal expansion was performed intraoperatively, postoperative flexible wires cannot prevent transverse relapse; In order for transverse control to be achieved, a palatal bar can be used (Winchester & Young, 2007).

The postoperative phase of the treatment needs to be completed within 4-5 months (Slavnic & Marcusson, 2010) after the operation, because mobilisation and cooperation on the part of patients dwindle after this period (Kiyak et al., 1984).

8. Retention

Retention is not different from that of usual orthodontic treatment for adult patients. So, dental movements achieved through preoperative and postoperative orthodontics, need a retention period that follows the removal of fixed appliances. This allows the alveolar bone and periodontal tissues to be reinforced. Where incisors' rotation has been corrected or large spaces closed, a fixed, stable, attached lingual or buccal retention mechanism is used. In other cases, a movable retention appliance may be used (Hunt, 2008b). When surgical or orthodontic expansion has been achieved, it should be maintained with retention for at least 1 year, because it is usually unstable (Phillips et al., 1992).

9. References

Arnett GW, Bergman RT. (1993a). Facial keys to orthodontic diagnosis and treatment planning. Part I. *American journal of orthodontics and dentofacial orthopedics*, Vol. 103, No. 4, pp. 299-312, ISSN 0889-5406.

Arnett GW, Bergman RT. (1993b). Facial keys to orthodontic diagnosis and treatment planning. Part II. *American journal of orthodontics and dentofacial orthopedics*, Vol. 103, No. 5, pp. 395-4ll, ISSN 0889-5406.

Athanasiou AE, Kragskov J. (1995). Computerized Cephalometric Systems. In: *Orthodontic Cephalometry*, Athanasiou AE, pp. 231-239, Mosby-Wolfe, ISBN 0 7234 2045 9, London.

Barber AF, Sims MR. (1981). Rapid maxillary expansion and external root resorption in man: a scanning electron microscope study. *American Journal of Orthodontics.* Vol. 79, No. 6, pp. 630-652, ISSN 0002-9416.

Bass NM. (1991). The aesthetic analysis of the face. *European Journal of Orthodontics*, Vol. 13, No. 5, pp. 343-50, ISSN 0141-5387.

Baumrind S, Frantz RC. (1971). The reliability of head film measurements. 1. Landmark identification. *American journal of orthodontics*, Vol. 60, No. 2, pp. 111-127, ISSN 0002-9416.

Boyd RL. (1978). Mucogingival considerations and their relationship to orthodontics. *Journaj of Periodontology*, Vol. 49, No 2, pp. 67-76, ISSN 0022-3492.

Burstone CJ. (1967). Lip posture and its significance in treatment planning. *American journal of orthodontics*, Vol. 53, No. 4, pp. 262-284, ISSN 0002-9416.

Chaconas SJ, Fragiskos FD. (1991). Orthognathic diagnosis and treatment planning: a cephalometric approach. *Journal of oral rehabilitation*, Vol. 18, No. 6, pp. 531-545, ISSN 0305-182X.

Chaconas SJ, Gonidis D (1986). A cephalometric technique for prosthodontic diagnosis and treatment planning. *The* Journal of Prosthetic Dentistry, Vol. 56, No. 5, pp. 567-74, ISSN 0022-3913.

Diaz PM, Garcia RG, Gias LN, Aguirre-Jaime A, Pérez JS, de la Plata MM, Navarro EV, Gonzalez FJ.(2010). Journal of Oral and Maxillofacial Surgery. Vol. 68, No. 1, pp. 88-92, ISSN 0278-2391.

Eales EA, Newton C, Jones ML, Sugar A. (1994). The accuracy of computerized prediction of the soft tissue profile: a study of 25 patients treated by means of the Le Fort I osteotomy. The *International Journal of Adult Orthodontics and Orthognathic Surgery*, Vol. 9, No. 2, 141-152, ISSN 0742-1931.

Fish LC, Epker BN. (1980). Surgical-orthodontic cephalometric prediction tracing. *Journal of clinical orthodontics*, Vol. 14, No. 1, pp. 36-52, ISSN 1079-5154.

Guariglia A, Ronchi P. (2005). Cephalometry in Dentofacial Anomalies, In: *Orthodontic-Surgical Treatment of Dentofacial Anomalies*, Ronchi P, pp. 35-45, Quintessenza, ISBN 88-7492-101-2, Milan Italy.

Harris M, Hunt N. (2008). General Assessment, In: *Fundamentals of Orthognathic Surgery*, Harris M, Hunt N, pp. 1-22, Imperial College Press, ISBN-13 978-1-86094-993-7, London UK.

Houston WJB. (1988). Mandibular growth rotations - their mechanisms and importance. European Journal of Orthodontics, Vol. 10, No. 4, pp. 369–373, ISSN 0141-5387.

Hunt N. (2008a). Radiographic Analysis and Imaging, In: *Fundamentals of Orthognathic Surgery*, Harris M, Hunt N, pp. 23-39, Imperial College Press, ISBN-13 978-1-86094-993-7, London UK.

Hunt N. (2008b). Orthodontic Preparation, In: *Fundamentals of Orthognathic Surgery*, Harris M, Hunt N, pp. 51-70, Imperial College Press, ISBN-13 978-1-86094-993-7, London UK.

Jacobs JD, Sinclair PM. (1983). Principles of orthodontic mechanics in orthognathic surgery cases. American journal of orthodontics. Vol. 84, No 5, pp. 399-407, ISSN 0002-9416.

Jensen AC, Sinclair PM, Wolford LM. (1992). Soft tissue changes associated with double jaw surgery. *American Journal of Orthodontist and Dentofacial Orthopedics*, Vol. 101, No. 3, pp. 266-275. ISSN 0889-5406.

Kaipatur NR, Flores-Mir C. (2009). Accuracy of computer programs in predicting orthognathic surgery soft tissue response. *Journal of Oral and Maxillofacial Surgery*. Vol. 67, No. 4, pp. 751-759. ISSN 0278-2391.

Kapila S, Conley RS, Harrell WE Jr. (2011). The current status of cone beam computed tomography imaging in orthodontics. *Dentomaxillofac Radiology*, Vol. 40, No. 1, pp. 24-34, . ISSN 0250-832X.

Kiyak HA, Hohl T, West RA, McNeil RW. (1984). Psychologic changes in orthognathic surgery patients: a 24 - month follow up. *Journal of Oral and Maxillofacial Surgery*, Vol. 42, No. 8, pp. 506-512, ISSN 0278-2391.

Kolokitha OE, Athanasiou AE, Tuncay O. (1996). Validity of computerized predictions of dentoskeletal and soft tissue profile changes after mandibular setback and maxillary impaction osteotomies. The *International Journal of Adult Orthodontics and Orthognathic Surgery*, Vol. 11, No. 2, pp. 137-154, ISSN 0742-1931.

Kolokitha OE. (2007). Validity of a manual soft tissue profile prediction method following mandibular setback osteotomy. *European Journal of Dental*, Vol. 1, No. 4, pp. 202-211. ISSN 0141-5387.

Lake SM, McNeill RW, Little RM, West RA. (1981). Surgical mandibular advancement: A cephalometric analysis of treatment response. *American journal of orthodontics*, Vol. 80, No. 4, pp. 376-394, ISSN 0002-9416.

Langlade M. (1981). *Diagnostic orthodontique*. Maloine S.A., ISBN 2-224-00738-8, Paris.

Langlade M. (1986). *Therapeutique orthodontique*. Maloine S.A., ISBN 2-224-00465-6, Paris.

Lee RT. (1994). The benefits of post-surgical orthodontic treatment. *British journal of orthodontics*. Vol. 21, No 3, pp. 265-74, ISSN:0301-228X.

Levander E, Malmgren O. (1988). Evaluation of the risk of root resorption during orthodontic treatment: a study of upper incisors. *European Journal of Orthodontics*, Vol. 10, No. 1, pp. 30-38, ISSN 0141-5387.

Lines PA, Lines RR, Lines C. (1978). Profilemetrics and facial esthetics. *American journal of orthodontics*, Vol. 73, No. 6, pp. 648-657, ISSN 0002-9416.

Liou EJ, Chen PH, Wang YC, Yu CC, Huang CS, Chen YR. (2011). Surgery-first accelerated orthognathic surgery: postoperative rapid orthodontic tooth movement. Journal of Oral and Maxillofacial Surgery. Vol.69, No.3, pp. 781-785, ISSN 0278-2391.

Luther F, Morris DO, Karnezi K. (2007). Orthodontic treatment following orthognathic surgery: how long does it take and why? A retrospective study. *Journal of Oral and Maxillofacial Surgery.* Vol.65, No.10, pp.1969-1976, ISSN 0278-2391.

McNamara JA. (1984). A method of cephalometric evaluation. *American journal of orthodontics,* Vol. 86, No. 6, pp. 449-469, ISSN 0002-9416.

McNamara JA, Brudon WL. (1993). Orthodontic and Orthopedic Treatment in the Mixed Dentition, pp. 13-54, Needham Press, ISBN 0-9635022-1-2, Ann Arbor USA.

McNamara JA, Ellis E. (1988). Cephalometric analysis of untreated adults with ideal facial and occlusal relationships. *The International journal of adult orthodontics and orthognathic surgery,* Vol. 3, No. 4, pp. 221-231, ISSN 0742-1931.

McNeill RW, Proffit WR, White RP. (1972). Cephalometric prediction for orthodontic surgery. The Angle orthodontist, Vol. 42, No. 2, pp. 154-164, ISSN 0003-3219.

Miethke R. (1995). Possibilities and Limitations of Various Cephalometric Variables and Analyses. In: *Orthodontic Cephalometry,* Athanasiou AE, pp. 63-103, Mosby-Wolfe, ISBN 0 7234 2045 9, London.

Muller L. (1962). *Cephalometrie et orthodontie,* SNPMD, ISBN 2-903482-06-3, Paris.

Onizawa K, Schmelzeisen R, Vogt S. (1995). Alteration of tem¬poromandibular joint symptoms after orthognathic sur¬gery: a comparison with healthy volunteers. Journal of oral and maxillofacial surgery, Vol. 53, No. 2, pp. 117-121, ISSN 0278-2391.

Phillips C, Medland WH, Fields HW, Profitt WR, White RP Jr. (1992). Stability of surgical maxillary expansion. The *International Journal of Adult Orthodontics and Orthognathic Surgery,* Vol. 7, No. 3, pp. 139-146, ISSN 0742-1931.

Proffit WR. (1991). Treatment planning: The search for wisdom. In: *Surgical Orthodontic Treatment.* Proffit WR, White RP Jr, pp. 142-191. Mosby, ISBN 0-8016-5291-X, St Louis USA.

Proffit WR, White RP Jr. (1991). Combined Surgical – Orthodontic Treatment: Who Does What, When?. In: *Surgical Orthodontic Treatment,* Proffit WR, White RP,Jr, pp. 192-224, Mosby, ISBN 0-8016-5291-X, St Louis USA.

Proffit WR, Fields HW. (1993). *Contemporary Orthodontics Second edition.* pp. 607-645, Mosby-Year Book, ISBN 0-8016-6393-8, St.Louis USA.

Proffit WR, Sarver DM. (2003). Treatment planning: Optimizing benefit to the patient. In: *Contemporary Treatment of Dentofacial Deformity.* Proffit WR, White RP,Jr, Sarver DM, pp. 172-244, Mosby, ISBN 0-323-01697-9, St.Louis USA.

Proffit WR, White RP, Jr. (2003). Combining Surgery and Orthodontics: Who Does What, When?. In: Contemporary Treatment of Dentofacial Deformity. Proffit WR, White RP,Jr, Sarver DM, pp. 245-267, Mosby, ISBN 0-323-01697-9, St.Louis USA.

Proffit WR, Fields HW. (2007). *Contemporary Orthodontics Fourth edition.* pp. 686-718, Mosby, ISBN 13: 978-0-323-04046-4, St.Louis USA.

Reyneke JP. (2003). *Essentials of Orthognathic Surgery*, Quintessence Publishing Co, ISBN 0-86715-410-1, China.

Ricketts RM, Roth RH, Chaconas SJ, Schulhof RJ, Engel GA. (1982). *Orthodontic diagnosis and planning Vol 1*, pp. 127-147, Rocky Mountain /Orthodontics, LCCN 82-62145, Denver, Colo. U.S.A.

Ricketts RM. (1975). A four-step method to distinguish orthodontic changes from natural growth. Journal of clinical orthodontics, Vol. 9, No. 4, pp. 208-28, ISSN 1079-5154.

Ricketts RM (1981). Perspectives in the clinical application of cephalometrics. The first fifty years. The Angle orthodontist, Vol. 51, No. 2, pp. 115-50, ISSN 0003-3219.

Sabri R. (2006). Orthodontic Objectives in Orthognathic surgery: state of the art today. *World Journal of Orthodontics*, Vol. 7, No. 2, pp. 177-191, ISSN 1530-5678.

Sassouni V (1958). Diagnosis and treatment planning via roentgenographic cephalometry. *American Journal of Orthodontist*, Vol. 44, No. 6, pp. 433-463, ISSN 0002-9416.

Sassouni V. (1971). *Orthodontics in dental practise*, Mosby, ISBN 8016-4300-7, St Louis USA.

Sinclair PM, Proffit WR. (1991). Class III Problems: Mandibular Excess - Maxillary Deficiency. In: *Surgical Orthodontic Treatment*, Proffit WR, White RP, pp. 428-482. Mosby, ISBN 0-8016-5291-X, St Louis USA.

Slavnic S, Marcusson A. (2010). Duration of orthodontic treatment in conjunction with orthognathic surgery. *Swedish Dental Journal*, Vol. 34, No. 3, pp. 159-166, ISSN 0347-9994.

Stroud LP. (1997). Mounted Study Casts and Cephalometric Analysis. In: *Science and Practice of Occlusion*, McNeill C, pp. 331-348, Quintessence Publishing Co, ISBN 9780867153040. Chicago USA.

Tompach PC, Wheeler JJ, Fridrich KL. (1995).Orthodontic considerations in orthognathic surgery. The *International Journal of Adult Orthodontics and Orthognathic Surgery*.Vol.10, No2, pp.97-107, ISSN 0742-1931.

Vion P. (1976). Anatomie teleradiographique en norma lateralis. *Revue d'Orthopédie Dento-Faciale*, Vol. 10, No. 4, pp. 449-537, ISSN 0337-9736.

Winchester LJ, Young DR. (2007). Orthodontic Role in Planning: Clinical Aspects, In: *Maxillofacial Surgery*, Booth PW, Schendel SA, Hausamen J-E, pp. 1211-1223, Churchill Livingstone Elsevier, ISBN-13 978-0-443-10053-6, St. Louis USA.

Wolford LM, Hilliard FW, Dugan DJ. (1985). *Surgical Treatment Objective. A Systematic Approach to the Prediction Tracing*, Mosby Year Book, ISBN 9780801656095, St Louis USA.

Wolford LM, Stevao ELL, Alexander CM, Goncalves JR. (2004). Orthodontics for Orthognathic Surgery, In: Peterson's Principals of Oral and Maxillofacial Surgery, Miloro M, Ghali GE, Larsen PE, Waite P, pp. 1111-1134, BC Decker Inc, ISBN 1-55009-234-0, Canada.

Wolford LM. (2007). Surgical Planning in Orthognathic Surgery, In: *Maxillofacial Surgery*, Booth PW, Schendel SA, Hausamen J-E, pp. 1155-1210, Churchill Livingstone Elsevier, ISBN-13 978-0-443-10053-6, St. Louis USA.

Worms FW, Isaacson RJ, Speidel TM. (1976). Surgical orthodontic treatment planning: prolile analysis and mandibular surgery. *The Angle orthodontist*, Vol. 46, No. 1, pp. 1-25, ISSN 0003-3219.

3

Long-Term Outcome of Orthognathic Surgery

Lisen Espeland and Arild Stenvik
University of Oslo
Norway

1. Introduction

Orthognathic surgery is treatment which often leads to great improvement in function and appearance, but is demanding to the patient, considerable resources are being spent, and risks for unwanted side effects are involved. Because of the elective nature of the treatment it is particularly important that the patient is well informed about all aspects of the provision and outcome of treatment before the decision to initiate treatment is reached. This information should be evidence-based. In this area it is, however, difficult to establish research materials that are both homogenous and of adequate size. The present chapter represents an attempt to summarize research findings from long-term follow-up of more than 1000 patients treated according to an established protocol over a period of 15 years.

2. Background

Since 1970 an orthognathic team of orthodontists and maxillofacial surgeons at the University of Oslo has monitored patients referred for advice and treatment planning, surgery, and a 3-year follow-up at regular intervals after the operation. The patient files comprise clinical recordings, photos, radiographs, and patient questionnaires. Cephalograms have been obtained 1 week before and 1 week, 2 and 6 months, and 1 and 3 years after surgery. The results presented here are based on observations from patients in whom the bony segments have been stabilized with rigid fixation only.

About 150 patients have been referred each year of whom 50 to 60% have undergone surgery. Pre-surgical orthodontic treatment lasts on average 18 months and post-surgical orthodontics 6 months (Dowling et al., 1999). The osteotomies that will be discussed in this chapter comprise one-piece LeFort I, bilateral sagittal split (BSSO) and extraoral vertical ramus osteotomies (EVRO), and genioplasty. Standardized protocols which have been followed over time have made it possible to establish homogenous subsamples of sufficient size for analyses of various aspects of treatment such as skeletal stability, sensory function, effect on airways and soft tissue profile, and patient satisfaction.

3. Stability

Skeletal relapse after orthognathic surgery may be due to biological factors like lack of neuromuscular adaptation and condylar resorption, as well as factors related to the surgical procedures. The extent of the relapse may be associated with the magnitude and direction of skeletal movements, the method of fixation, and the use of bone grafts. A hierarchy of stability based on initial anatomy and various surgical procedures has been proposed (Proffit et al., 1996). Relapse may be presented as the mean post-surgical change, or as the rate of subjects with a clinically significant relapse, usually defined as change of 2 mm or more. Another issue of importance is when the relapse occurs, and hence short- and long-term stability should be examined. Skeletal relapse may also to a varying extent impact on occlusal stability.

3.1 Skeletal stability

The results presented below is a compilation of findings from studies performed at the University of Oslo. The cephalometric variables have been recorded as x- and y-coordinates (Fig. 1). The x-axis was constructed 7° to the nasion-sella line. The most common osteotomies for management of Class II and III skeletal malocclusions will be addressed.

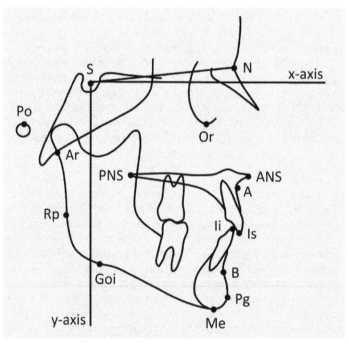

Fig. 1. Cephalometric landmarks used in analyses of stability

3.1.1 Class III: mandibular setback

The bilateral sagittal split osteotomy (BSSO) is a versatile and widely used approach for correction of mandibular prognathism. In a study of 80 (46 males, 34 females) consecutively operated patients (Mobarak et al., 2000a) this procedure appeared to be fairly stable. Three years post-surgery the mean relapse was 1.6 mm and represented 26% of the surgical setback at Pogonion (Pg) (6.3 mm). In 36% of the patients relapse was clinically significant (≥ 2 mm). Most of the relapse took place during the first 6 months after surgery (72%) (Fig. 2). The magnitude of the setback was to some extent associated with the amount of horizontal relapse (r = 0.39, P < 0.01). Gender differences in relapse were small.

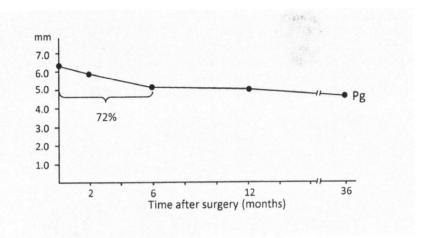

Fig. 2. Mean postsurgical horizontal change at Pg as a function of time in 80 mandibular setback (BSSO) patients.

An alternative approach to BSSO is the vertical ramus osteotomy (VRO). Traditionally the VRO has required intermaxillary fixation for 6-8 weeks. Since 1995, stable plate fixation has routinely been used with an extraoral incision by our team (Hoegevold et al., 2001) (Fig. 3). The main morphologic indication for applying the extraoral VRO (EVRO) has been a moderate setback without rotation. Another indication is related to reduced risk for sensory disturbances. In a 1-year follow-up study post-operative changes were mainly in the form of a small anterior relapse tendency of about 10% of the surgical setback. Mean relapse was 0.6 mm (SD 1.2 mm). A relapse ≥ 2 mm was observed in 14% of the subjects (Mobarak et al., 2000b).

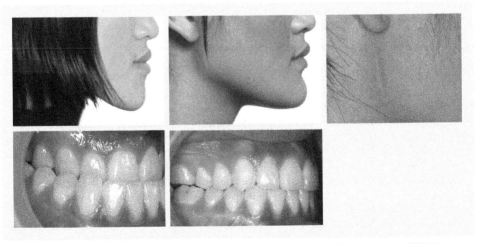

Fig. 3. Patient with mandibular prognathism before treatment and 3 years after EVRO. Facial scar after extraoral incision to the right.

3.1.2 Class III: maxillary advancement

After the LeFort I osteotomy became common in the 1970-ies, this is an increasingly used alternative to correct Class III malocclusion. This approach allows treatment based on the diagnosis in cases where the discrepancy is caused by a retrognathic maxilla (Fig. 4). In addition to be associated with few unwanted side-effects like nerve injuries, a negative impact on the airways which may occur after mandibular setback, is avoided.

In a sample of 43 individuals having had maxillary advancement of ≥ 2 mm (mean advancement 5 mm), the mean relapse was 0.9 mm (18%), and the relapse was clinically significant in 14% of the patients (Dowling et al., 2005). Almost all (89%) of the relapse took place during the first 6 months. Regression analysis identified large advancements and downward movement of the anterior maxilla as risk factors for horizontal relapse.

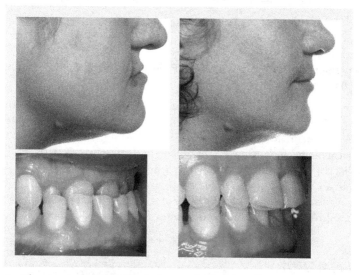

Fig. 4. Patient with retrognathic maxilla before and after maxillary advancement (one-piece LeFort I).

3.1.3 Class III: bimaxillary surgery

In patients with severe skeletal discrepancies single jaw surgery may not be possible or may have an unwanted effect on the patient's facial appearance. In later years, there has been a trend for increased use of a combination of mandibular setback and maxillary advancement. Severe skeletal Class III malocclusions are frequently associated with anterior open bite, which is more readily corrected with bimaxillary surgery and may also ensure optimal facial harmony (Fig. 5).

A study of stability comprised 81 patients (Jakobsone et al., 2011a) who pre-surgery had a mean negative overjet of -7 mm (range -18.9 to 3.2 mm) and a negative overbite of -1.8 (range -9.7 to 6.4 mm). Skeletal stability assessed 3 years after surgery varied depending on the direction and amount of the surgical repositioning. Maxillary advancement was stable, whereas a significant mean relapse was observed after mandibular setback (Fig. 6). About half of the 62 subjects with a setback of 2 mm or more, had a clinically significant relapse. Most of the skeletal relapse occurred during the first 6 months after surgery. Regression analysis showed that stability was increased when the setback was small and the posterior maxilla was impacted.

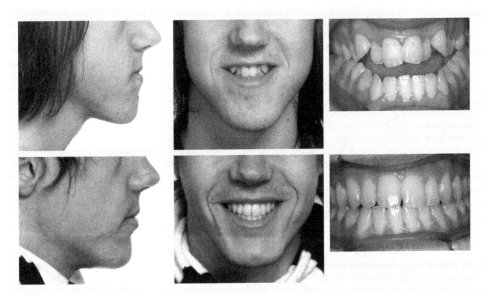

Fig. 5. Patient with severe Class III malocclusion and open bite corrected with one-piece LeFort I and BSSO (before treatment and 3 years after surgery).

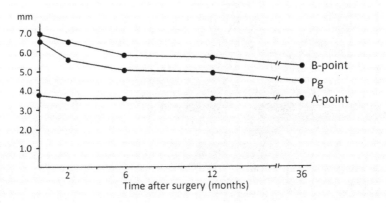

Fig. 6. Mean horizontal changes at various cephalometric landmarks as a function of time in 81 Class III patients having bimaxillary surgery (BSSO and one-piece LeFort I).

3.1.4 Class II: mandibular advancement

The BSSO is the most frequently used osteotomy for management of mandibular retrognatism. High-angle and low-angle Class II cases represent two distinct entities, with different facial patterns, treatment goals, and clinical challenges.

A study of stability analysed these two categories separately in 61 consecutive cases (Mobarak et al., 2001a). High- (n = 20) and low-angle (n = 20) patients had different patterns of surgical and post-operative skeletal changes. High-angle cases were associated with greater horizontal relapse. Relapse in the low-angle cases occurred early in the post-operative period, whereas in the high-angle cases, relapse was a more continuous process with a significant proportion occurring later in the follow-up period (Fig. 7). Increasing the anterior facial height (low-angle) was a relatively stable procedure, with on average 70% of the improvement remaining after 3 years.

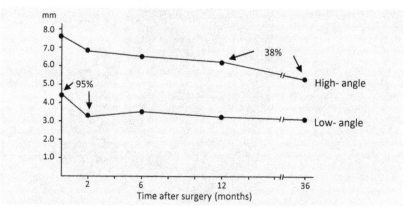

Fig. 7. Mean horizontal changes at Pg in low- and high-angle cases as a function of time. Mean surgical advancement appears from the vertical axis.

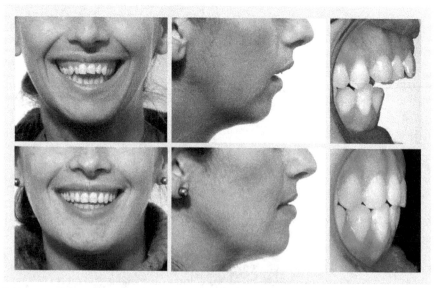

Fig. 8. Patient with severe Class II with open bite and high-angle facial pattern before treatment and 3 years after surgery with BSSO and one-piece LeFort I.

3.1.5 Class II: bimaxillary surgery

Our studies of stability after bimaxillary surgery to correct skeletal Class II malocclusion have focused on subjects with a high-angle facial pattern as this group represents the greatest challenge. In a study of 31 patients (ML/NSL > 38°) the stability of maxillary impaction and mandibular advancement varied considerably (Winter et al., 2010). Stable results (relapse < 2 mm) after maxillary impaction were observed in 77% of the subjects, whereas mandibular advancements were stable in only 42%. Despite the risk for relapse, some patients showed excellent results after 3 years (Fig. 8).

3.1.6 Class II: advancement genioplasty

Genioplasty allows 3-dimensional control of chin position, resulting in significant improvement of facial aesthetics whether performed separately or combined with other osteotomies. Of the actual corrections of the chin, advancement genioplasty to improve a receding chin is probably the most common.

Our study of stability after advancement genioplasty included 21 subjects who had no additional osteotomies (Shaughnessy et al., 2006) (Fig. 9). Mean advancement was 8.4 mm. The results 3 years after surgery showed that this was a stable procedure with a mean relapse of only 8% of the advancement. Some of the post-surgical change could be ascribed to remodelling in the area rather than instability of the segment.

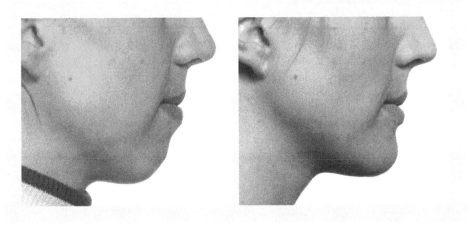

Fig. 9. Advancement genioplasty patient pre-treatment (left) and 3 years after surgery (right).

3.1.7 Open bite correction by isolated maxillary surgery

Open bite occurs both in Class I, II, and III malocclusions. When the sagittal discrepancy is moderate, the occlusion can usually be corrected by LeFort I impaction as the only procedure (Fig. 10). In a study of 40 consecutively operated patients (Espeland et al., 2008a) it was observed that impaction of posterior maxilla (≥ 2 mm) relapsed by one third. Inferior movement of the anterior maxilla relapsed about two thirds. Most of the relapse occurred during the first 6 months after surgery.

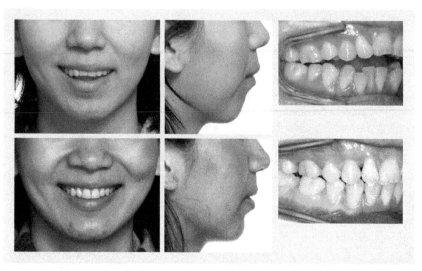

Fig. 10. Patient with open bite before treatment and after one-piece LeFort I with impaction of posterior maxilla.

3.1.8 Summary – skeletal stability

Fig. 11 summarizes frequencies of stable results (relapse < 2 mm) after various one-jaw osteotomies. The most stable results were observed after advancement of the maxilla, setback of the mandible (EVRO), and advancement of the chin. The least stable procedures were advancement of the mandible in patients with high-angle facial pattern and downward movement of the maxilla. In the literature a number of factors have been proposed which may explain skeletal relapse. For Class III anomalies early relapse has been associated with clockwise rotation of the proximal segment during BSSO-surgery (Proffit et al., 1996). In our study (Mobarak et al., 2000a), however, this did not seem to be responsible for marked relapse. Late relapse has often been ascribed to late mandibular growth which our findings also indicated. For Class II corrections by BSSO advancement, early relapse has been suggested to be due to suboptimal positioning of the condyle, whereas condylar resorption might be responsible for relapse occurring later. Risk factors for condylar resorption have been addressed in the literature, for example condylar morphology and bone quality (Hoppenreijs et al., 1999).

3.2 Occlusal stability

Despite some skeletal relapse after most surgical corrections, the anterior occlusion is generally stable. In the studies addressing stability referred to above, the incisor relationship was also examined. Below is a short summary of the main findings.

After Class III correction by one-jaw surgery, both with setback of the mandible (Mobarak et al., 2000a) and advancement of the maxilla (Dowling et al., 2005), all patients examined had a positive overjet 3 years after the operation. Bimaxillary surgery resulted in positive overjet in 79 of 81 patients (Jakobsone et al., 2011a). Relapse of open bite was observed in 8 subjects, and in 5 of these, the negative overbite was less than 1 mm.

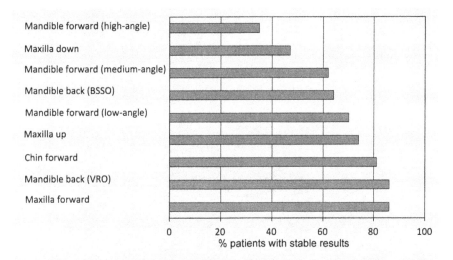

Fig. 11. Diagrammatic representation of stability after various one-jaw surgical procedures. Bars represent frequency of patients with relapse less than 2 mm 3 years after surgery.

After Class II correction with mandibular advancement, the difference in skeletal stability between patients with low- and high-angle facial pattern was reflected in the stability of the occlusion. After 3 years 85% of the low-angle patients had overjet less than 4 mm, whereas the corresponding figure for the high-angle subjects was 60%. In the group of 41 high-angle patients treated with bimaxillary surgery, one third of those having overjet > 6 mm before surgery, still had an overjet > 6 mm after 3 years.

Of 40 open-bite patients treated by isolated LeFort I impaction, 88% had positive overbite 3 years post-surgery (Espeland et al., 2008a). In all the remaining patients, the negative overbite was less than 1 mm. The skeletal relapse was counteracted by dentoalveolar compensation, which contributed to approximately 50% of the correction of the overbite.

For all categories of malocclusion, the skeletal relapse generally took place during the first 6 months. A negative effect on the occlusion was avoided for most patients by dentoalveolar compensation, which underlines the importance of post-surgical monitoring and orthodontic management if signs of relapse become apparent.

4. Soft tissue response

Software for prediction of the soft tissue response has become an integral part of treatment planning aiming to provide a realistic estimate of the outcome of surgery. Ratios (or percentages) for soft to hard tissue changes have focused in particular on nose, lips, mentolabial fold, and chin. It is important that the data which serve to generate software prediction programs are valid. Changes in sagittal and vertical dimensions as well as lip thickness have been addressed in studies at our department.

4.1 Class III: mandibular setback
The soft tissue response for the lower lip, mentolabial fold and soft tissue chin to the underlying hard tissues was about 1:1. Some effect was also seen for the upper lip (Fig. 12).

The main effect of mandibular setback on the soft tissue profile included an increase in facial convexity, straightening and lengthening of the upper lip with a concomitant increase in nasolabial angle, and deepening of the mentolabial fold (Mobarak et al., 2001b).

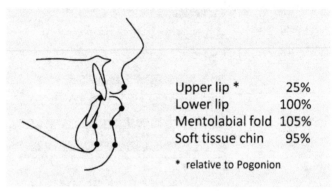

Upper lip *   25%
Lower lip   100%
Mentolabial fold 105%
Soft tissue chin   95%

* relative to Pogonion

Fig. 12. Relationship between soft and hard tissue horizontal changes after mandibular setback in 80 patients (BSSO).

4.2 Class III: bimaxillar surgery
To quantify the relative soft tissue response to the skeletal changes, a sample of 80 patients were divided in 3 subgroups according to pre-operative characteristics: 1) open bite, 2) positive overbite and the upper lip resting on upper incisors, and 3) positive overbite and the upper lip resting on lower incisors (lip block) (Jakobsone et al., 2011b).
In the first two groups, there were strong correlations between the horizontal movement of upper incisors and upper lip (r = 0.77 and 0.85, respectively). The upper lip followed the maxilla with a ratio of 0.5:1. When the upper lip rested on lower incisors before surgery, the association between maxillary repositioning and upper lip changes were weak. In all groups a strong association between horizontal soft and hard tissue changes of lower lip and chin was observed. The vertical position of the tip of the nose was affected by both the vertical and horizontal repositioning of the maxilla. Several factors influencing the soft tissue response were identified. Software prediction programs should preferably take into account different pre-surgical characteristics.

4.3 Class II: mandibular advancement
The ratio for the soft to hard tissue response after mandibular advancement was about 1:1 for the chin and 0.6:1 for the lower lip. For the mentolabial fold, the ratio was on average 0.9:1, but varied somewhat according to vertical facial pattern (Mobarak et al., 2001c). Following mandibular advancement the facial profile became straighter. The mentolabial fold became more shallow, especially in low-angle subjects who also had an increase in anterior facial height.

4.4 Class II: advancement genioplasty
In our study of soft tissue response to advancement of the chin as the only surgical procedure, the results showed that the ratio for soft to hard tissue movement was 0.9:1 (Shaughnessy et al., 2006). The mentolabial depth increased as a result of treatment (Fig. 9).

5. Effect on upper airways

In addition to the changes in masticatory function and facial harmony, repositioning of the jaws may also impact on airway morphology. Mandibular advancement and setback osteotomies have been reported to influence the position of the hyoid bone, and consequently tongue position, pharyngeal airway morphology, and head flexion (Achilleos et al., 2000a,b). Studies have also shown that in adults, there is on average a reduction in the sagittal dimension of the minimal pharyngeal airway space with increasing age (Kollias & Krogstad, 1999). Over the last two decades the capacity of maxillo-mandibular osteotomies to induce or resolve obstructive sleep apnoea (OSA) has received increased attention. A challenge in the planning of orthognathic surgery is to balance concerns related to facial aesthetics and airway changes.

A recent study of bimaxillary correction of Class III malocclusion examined whether maxillary advancement and/or impaction had the potential to compensate for the negative effect of mandibular setback on airways (Jakobsone et al., 2011c).

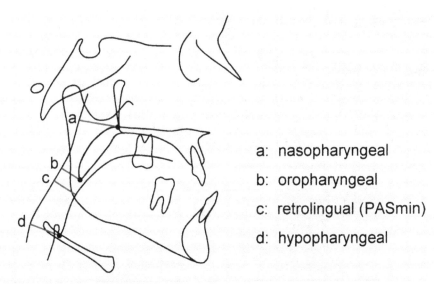

a: nasopharyngeal

b: oropharyngeal

c: retrolingual (PASmin)

d: hypopharyngeal

Fig. 13. The 4 levels in the upper airways which were cephalometrically examined.

Sagittal dimensions of the pharynx were measured on 4 different levels (Fig. 13) in 4 subgroups. The long-term change (3 years) at the various levels related to whether the maxilla was advanced and/or impacted or not, appears from Fig. 14. Advancement of the maxilla resulted in an increase of 15-20% at the nasopharyngeal level. At the hypopharyngeal level, advancement of the maxilla did to some extent compensate for the negative effect of mandibular setback. A decrease of 5-10% was observed at the oropharyngeal and retrolingual (PASmin) levels.

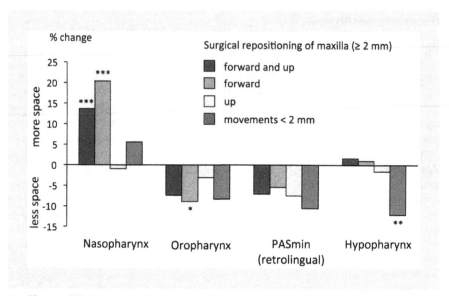

Fig. 14. Change (%) in sagittal dimension of the upper airways related to varying maxillary repositionings in subjects undergoing bimaxillary surgery for correction of Class III malocclusion.

6. Sensory function

Impairment of sensory function is the most common long-term side effect after orthognathic surgery, especially following sagittal split osteotomies (Westermark et al., 1999). In our sample of 381 patients operated with bilateral sagittal split osteotomy (BSSO), 47.8% reported altered sensory function 3 years after the operation (Table 1).

Patient's report	% patients
Normal /almost normal	52.2
Reduced	40.4
Increased	6.3
Complete loss	1.0

Table 1. Patients' reports of sensation in the lower lip and chin 3 years after bilateral sagittal split osteotomy.

Among patients with impaired sensation (n=181), 40.9% indicated that the impairment was of concern to them because it affected their daily life. A mild distress was reported by 28.2%, 8.3% reported a moderate distress, and 4.4% said the situation caused severe distress. The age at the time of surgery was significantly associated with self-reported alterations in sensory function ($P < 0.001$). Distress due to impaired sensation also increased with age ($P = 0.024$) (Fig. 15).

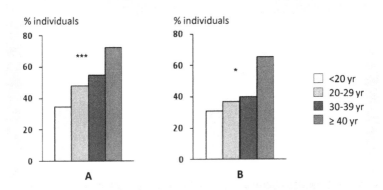

Fig. 15. **A:** Relative frequency of individuals reporting altered sensory function according to age among 381 subjects operated with BSSO. **B:** Relative frequency of individuals reporting varying levels of distress (mild, moderate, and severe combined) according to age among 181 who reported altered sensation. * P < 0.05, *** P < 0.001.

7. Patients' satisfaction with treatment results

Orthognathic surgery may have an impact on quality of life (Cunningham et al., 2002). At a clinical review 3 years after surgery, patients monitored by our team fill in a questionnaire addressing their opinions of the treatment result in terms of improvement in dental and facial appearance, chewing ability, speech, impact on social life, satisfaction with overall result, and whether they would re-elect surgery with their present experience (Espeland et al., 2008b). Findings among 705 consecutively operated patients appear from Tables 2–4. Totally 90.6% reported that they were satisfied with the overall treatment result, and 88.5% indicated that they would have re-elected surgery based on their present experiences. Of those expressing dissatisfaction, 47.0% stated that they would have made the same decision.

	Very satisfied	Satisfied	Somewhat dissatisfied	Very dissatisfied
Females (n=399)	56.6	31.1	10.5	1.8
Males (n=306)	64,4	30.1	4.9	0.7
Total (n=705)	60.0	30.6	8.1	1.3

Table 2. Patients' answers to a question about satisfaction with the treatment result (%). Significant difference between genders ($P = 0.017$).

	Satisfied (%)	Dissatisfied (%)
Skeletal Class I (n=97)	93.8	6.2
Skeletal Class II (n=214)	82.2	17.8
Skeletal Class III (n=394)	94.4	5.6

Table 3. Patients' reports on satisfaction/dissatisfaction related to skeletal malocclusion. Significant difference between categories ($P < 0.001$).

	Satisfied (%)	Dissatisfied (%)
Mandibular setback (n=226)	96.0	4.0
Mandibular setback and LeFort I (n=119)	94.1	5.9
Mandibular advancement (n=130)	83.1	16.9
Mandibular advancement and LeFort I (n=30)	76.7	23.3
Maxillary surgery (LeFort I) (n=124)	88.7	11.3
Other procedures (n=76)	90.8	9.2

Table 3. Patients' reports on satisfaction/dissatisfaction related to surgical approach. Significant difference between approaches (P < 0.001).

Relatively more males than females were satisfied, and correction of Class III malocclusion was associated with increased frequency of satisfied patients. The patients' stated reasons for dissatisfaction were allocated to the following categories: impaired nerve function (n=16), relapse (n=18), appearance (n=17), TMJ problems (n=8), occlusal function (6), and other reasons (n=11).

8. Concluding remarks

Orthognatic surgery may on the basis of systematic monitoring of outcomes according to our established protocols be regarded as a treatment modality that predictably leads to the correction of severe occlusal anomalies. Skeletal corrections are also generally stable and even if some relapse may occur, the occlusion is usually not affected due to orthodontic compensation during the first post-surgical months. Most patients are also satisfied with the result. Improvement in facial soft-tissue profile and the effect on upper airways are less predictable. Class II malocclusions represents a greater challenge compared to other anomalies, especially in patients with high-angle facial pattern.

9. Acknowledgment

The authors are greatly indebted to Håkon Størmer for excellent support in preparation of the illustrations.

10. References

Achilleos, S., Krogstad, O. & Lyberg T. (1979). Surgical mandibular advancement and changes in uvuloglossopharyngeal morphology and head posture : a short- and long-term cephalometric study in males. European Journal of Orthodontics, Vol.22, No.4, (August 2000a), pp. 367-381, ISSN 0141-5387

Achilleos, S., Krogstad, O. & Lyberg T. (1979). Surgical mandibular setback and changes in uvuloglossopharyngeal morphology and head posture : a short- and long-term cephalometric study in males. European Journal of Orthodontics, Vol.22, No.4, (August 2000b), pp. 383-394, ISSN 0141-5387

Cunningham S.J., Garratt, A.M. & Hunt, M.P. (1973). Development of a condition-specific quality of life measure for patients with dentofacial deformity: II. Validity and responsiveness testing. Community Dentistry and Oral Epidemiology, Vol.30, No.2, (April 2002), pp. 81-90, ISSN 0301-5661

Dowling, P.A., Espeland, L., Krogstad, O., Stenvik, A. & Kelly, A. (1986). Duration of orthodontic treatment involving orthognathic surgery. *The International Journal of Adult Orthodontics and Orthognathic Surgery*, Vol. 14, No.2, (Summer 1999), pp. 146-152, ISSN 0742-1931

Dowling, P.A., Espeland, L., Mobarak, K.A. & Hogevold, H.E. (1986). LeFort I maxillary advancement: 3-year stability and risk factors for relapse. *American Journal of Orthodontics and Dentofacial Orthopedics*, Vol.128, No.5 (November 2005), pp. 560-567, ISSN 0889-5406

Espeland, L., Dowling, P.A., Mobarak, K.A. & Stenvik, A. (1986). Three-year stability of open-bite correction by 1-piece maxillary osteotomy. *American Journal of Orthodontics and Dentofacial Orthopedics*, Vol.134, No.1, (July 2008a), pp. 60-66, ISSN 0889-5406

Espeland, L., Høgevold H.E. & Stenvik, A. (1979). A 3-year patient-centred follow-up of 516 consecutively treated orthognathic surgery patients. *European Journal of Orthodontics*, Vol.30, No.1, (February 2008b), pp. 24-30, ISSN 0141-5387

Hoppenreijs, T.J.M., Stoelinga, P.J.W., Grace, K.L. & Robben, C.M.G. (1986). Long-term evaluation of patients with progressive condylar resorption following orthognathic surgery. *International Journal of Oral and Maxillofacial Surgery*, Vol.28, No.6, (December 1999), pp. 411-418, ISSN 0901-5027

Høgevold, H.E., Mobarak, K.A., Espeland, L., Krogstad, O. & Skjelbred, P. (1987). Plate fixation of extra-oral subcondylar ramus osteotomy for correction of mandibular prognathism: clinical aspects and short term stability. *Journal of Cranio-maxillo-facial Surgery*, Vol.29, No.4, (August 2001), pp. 205-211, ISSN 1010-5182

Jakobsone, G., Stenvik A., Sandvik, L. & Espeland, L. (1986). Three-year follow-up of bimaxillary surgery to correct skeletal Class III malocclusion: stability and risk factors for relapse. *American Journal of Orthodontics and Dentofacial Orthopedics*, Vol.139, No.1, (January 2011a), pp. 80-89, ISSN 0889-5406

Jakobsone, G., Stenvik, A. & Espeland, L. Predicting the soft tissue profile changes after bimaxillary operations for Class III correction, *Proceedings of EOS 2011 87th Congress of the European Orthodontic Society*, Istanbul, Turkey, June 19-23, 2011b

Jakobsone, G., Stenvik, A. & Espeland, L. (1986). The effect of maxillary advancement and impaction on the upper airway after bimaxillary surgery to correct Class III malocclusion. *American Journal of Orthodontics and Dentofacial Orthopedics*, (April 2011c) (in press)

Kollias, I. & Krogstad, O. (1979). Adult craniocervical and pharyngeal changes – a longitudinal cephalometric study between 22 and 42 years of age. Part II: morphological uvulo-glossopharyngeal changes. *European Journal of Orthodontics*, Vol.21, No.4, (August 1999), pp. 345-355, ISSN 0141-5387

Mobarak, K.A., Krogstad, O., Espeland, L. & Lyberg, T. (1986). Long-term stability of mandibular setback surgery: a follow-up of 80 bilateral sagittal split osteotomy patients. *The International Journal of Adult Orthodontics and Orthognathic Surgery*, Vol 15, No.2, (Summer 2000a), pp. 83-95, ISSN 0742-1931

Mobarak, K.A., Krogstad, O., Espeland, L. & Lyberg, T. (1986). Stability of extraoral vertical ramus osteotomy: plate fixation versus maxillomandibular/skeletal suspension wire fixation. *The International Journal of Adult Orthodontics and Orthognathic Surgery*, Vol.15, No.2, (Summer 2000b), pp. 97-113, ISSN 0742-1931

Mobarak, K.A., Espeland, L., Krogstad, O. & Lyberg, T. (1986). Mandibular advancement surgery in high-angle and low-angle Class II patients: different long-term skeletal responses. *American Journal of Orthodontics and Dentofacial Orthopedics*, Vol.119, No.4, (April 2001a), pp. 368-381, ISSN 0889-5406

Mobarak, K.A., Krogstad, O., Espeland, L. & Lyberg, T. (1931). Factors influencing the predictability of soft tissue profile changes following mandibular setback surgery. *The Angle Orthodontist*, Vol.71, No.3, (June 2001b), pp. 216-227, ISSN 0003-3219

Mobarak, K.A., Espeland, L., Krogstad, O. & Lyberg, T. (1986). Soft tissue profile changes following mandibular advancement surgery: predictability and long-term outcome. *American Journal of Orthodontics and Dentofacial Orthopedics*, Vol.119, No.4, (April 2001c), pp. 353-367, ISSN 0889-5406

Proffit, W.R., Turvey, T.A. & Phillips, C. (1986). Orthognathic surgery: A hierarchy of stability. *The International Journal of Adult Orthodontics and Orthognathic Surgery*, Vol.11, No.3 (1996), pp. 191-204, ISSN 0742-1931

Shaughnessy, S., Mobarak, K.A., Høgevold, H.E. & Espeland L. (1986). Long-term skeletal and soft-tissue responses after advancement genioplasty. *American Journal of Orthodontics and Dentofacial Orthopedics*, Vol.130, No.1. (July 2006), pp. 8-17, ISSN 0889-5406

Westermark, A., Bystedt, H. & von Konow, L. (1986). Patients' evaluation of the final result of sagittal split osteotomy: is it influenced by impaired sensitivity of the lower lip and chin? *The International Journal of Adult Orthodontics and Orthognathic Surgery*, Vol.14, No.2, (Summer 1999), pp. 135-139, ISSN 0742-1931

Winter, B.U., Stenvik, A. & Espeland, L. Bimaxillary orthognathic surgery of high-angle skeletal Class II malocclusions – stability after 3 years, *Proceedings of WFO 2010 7th International Orthodontic Congress*, Sydney, Australia, Abstract 1505, February 6-9, 2010

4

Surgical Orthodontic Treatment of Class III Malocclusions

Paolo Ronchi[1] and Alberto Guariglia[2]

[1]*Maxillo-Facial Unit, St. Anna Hospital, Como,*
[2]*Private Practice, Milan,*
Italy

1. Introduction

The correction of dental malocclusions has always had a dual goal, functional and aesthetic. Normal stomatognathic functioning associated with satisfactory facial aesthetics must inevitably have significant repercussions on a patient's general state of health. The physical health of patients with severe malocclusion may be altered or compromised in various ways; if the problem is such as to significantly reduce masticatory capability there may be repercussions on the digestive tract or, in some cases, impossibility of chewing certain types of food. Marked dentoskeletal malposition may cause problems with speech or induce respiratory deficiency in the upper airways.

If teeth are irregular, protruded or crowded it is more difficult to maintain good oral hygiene, with a consequent increased predisposition to caries, and periodontal problems may become severe. Some conditions also predispose to an increased probability of developing temporomandibular joint pain and/or dysfunction (Laskin et al 1986, White & Dolwich, 1992).

Nevertheless, we believe that the aesthetic aspect of severe malocclusion with its related psycho-social impact is more important than the correlated physical problems, above all in modern society. The positive effect of having an attractive face on an individual's mind-frame are clear, in terms of self confidence and self respect; and on the other hand it is quite probable that a subject with a severe dentoskeletal alteration may develop such a significant lack of self-confidence, or even depression of varying severity. Thus the cornerstone for valid treatment must be to combine good functionality and satisfactory aesthetics.

In recent years, increasing numbers of patients elect to undergo orthodontic-surgical treatment to correct severe malocclusion not susceptible to simple orthodontic solution: currently this type of alteration is defined as dentofacial anomaly or dentofacial deformity.

But who should be given orthodontic-surgical treatment in class III patients? The most immediate and the simplest reply to this question, but also the most banal one, is that orthodontic-surgical treatment is necessary whenever orthodontics alone is insufficient to resolve the problem. In reality, this response is both inexact and insufficient, and furthermore it conceals a severe risk: that of beginning exclusive orthodontic treatment only to realize, after treatment is underway, the impossibility of achieving a good final result. This may leave the patient in a dramatic and irreversible situation. Thus the response must be both more complete and more complex (Ronchi, 2005).

In cases of severe malocclusion with dentoskeletal discrepancy there are generally only three possible therapeutic options: modification of growth; camouflage through dental compensation; surgical repositioning of the bony bases.

With regard to growth, it is obvious that the fundamental parameters we must consider are age, gender, type of malocclusion and skeletal involvement in the defect. Clearly, age and gender impose precise limits with regard to the timing of any orthopedic-functional treatment. Furthermore, at present there is reasonable consensus on two fundamental points. Firstly, growth may be modified favorably only in some types of patient, which rather limits this approach: the maxilla or the mandible may be stimulated to grow by a few additional millimeters (much more difficult to limit growth by the same amount) than would have occurred naturally. Thus it is not possible to obtain significant transformations. Secondly, during all orthopedic-functional treatment the teeth inevitably also move in the direction of the correct occlusal relation. This tooth movement, which may be called "dental compensation for skeletal discrepancies" hinders complete orthopedic-skeletal correction and introduces some elements of dental camouflage.

In our view, we may deduce from these considerations, for example, that in Class III, orthopedic treatment only plays a role in cases of slight isolated maxillary hypodevelopment with no mandibular protrusion and without any significant vertical alteration. In all other cases treatment should be postponed until the end of growth, when surgical correction will be applied.

Concerning the purely orthodontic treatment, with regard to subjects in whom growth is complete, it is clear that there is a lot of contingent difficulties relating to tooth movement: periodontal conditions, bone support, morphological and structural characteristics of the alveolar bone in which the teeth must move, patient collaboration and compliance. Furthermore, these camouflage corrections, even if possible from the theoretical and technical standpoints, are not always associated with improvement in facial aesthetics. In reality dental camouflage only leads to an effective improvement of aesthetics in a few situations. More frequently it has no significant influence on facial aesthetics, as in purely orthodontic correction of Class III cases.

We are now in a position to give a rather more complete reply to the above question: in a subject during growth, malocclusion may be considered too severe to be corrected without the help of surgery when the changes to growth that can be achieved with dentofacial orthopedics for that type of condition are not sufficient to ensure an optimal result from the functional and aesthetic standpoints. In an adult with dentoskeletal discrepancy, surgery is the only sure treatment option if the dental defect cannot be corrected by orthodontics alone or if dental camouflage would involve technical or periodontal contraindications, or would not produce a marked aesthetic improvement (Ronchi, 2005).

We may therefore reasonably say that the great majority of adult Class III patients require orthodontic-surgical treatment, chiefly in order to provide an optimal solution to their aesthetic problems.

Lastly, we must consider that the improvement that has come about in surgical techniques over recent years has undoubtedly helped to decrease surgery-related complications and to improve patients' post-operative progress. We may therefore assume that indications to orthodontic-surgical treatment of dentoskeletal discrepancies will continue to increase, above all in the interest of patients. However, we must not forget that all such treatment is always elective, though it is also in part therapeutic and in part preventive; that it involves at the same time and with equal importance both aesthetics and functionality; and that fundamentally it must contribute to improving the quality of life for our patients from the psychological and physical standpoints. This is the approach and the philosophy that must always guide the physician in his or her work and in his or her treatment choices.

2. Clinical features

Clinical examination of a patient with Class III malocclusion, as indeed with all types of dentofacial anomaly, must be extremely thorough; it must analyze occlusion and, above all, must carefully evaluate the morphological characteristics of the face. This type of anomaly cannot and must not only be examined in the sagittal direction, since frequently transverse or vertical alterations exist that are so significant as to influence the treatment plan. Clinical examination of the face takes time and is of particular importance. The face should be evaluated from the front, in profile and in three-quarters profile (Figure 1,2,3,4,5).

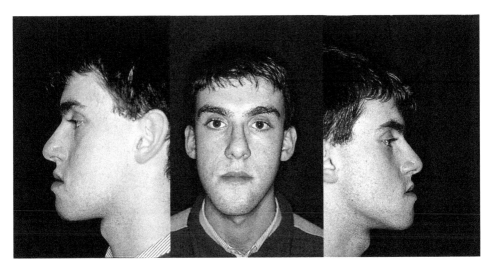

Figs. 1, 2, 3. Front and profile (left and right) of the patient

For simplicity data may be transcribed onto the medical record only for the frontal view and profile, but the evaluation must always be as complete as possible (we must remember that the patient always sees him or herself from the front or in three-quarters profile, almost never in profile!). The clinical examination should begin from the top, proceeding from forehead to neck. The following should be considered: hairline, frontal eminences, palpebral fissures, intercanthal distance, prominence or otherwise of the cheek-bones, thickness of the cheeks and of the soft tissues in general. Particular attention must be paid in these patients to the sub-orbital area, also evaluating the characteristics of the infraorbital rim and determining the presence or otherwise of scleral exposure on looking forwards (Figure 6).

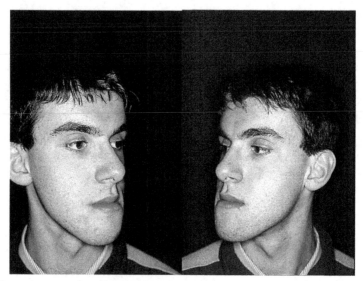

Figs. 4, 5. Three quarter view of the patient (right and left)

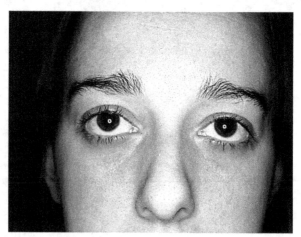

Fig. 6. Tipical example of scleral show

The nose, the central structure of the face, is of great importance in the clinical examination: glabella, dorsum, hump if any, characteristics of the tip, the columella and the opening of the nares should all be carefully examined. The width of the alar base should be measured, both the maximum distance and that at the point of insertion on the upper lip, and their mobility during speech and smiling should also be observed. Lastly, anterior rhinoscopy can reveal any deviation of the septum and the presence of endonasal synechia. The lips must also be examined both at rest and in movement, evaluating shape, thickness and muscle tone, as well as the shape and characteristics of the prolabium and of the Cupid's bow, any hypertrophism of the frenulae, labial competence or incompetence (obviously this is evaluated with the lips completely relaxed with no contraction, see Figure 7,8).

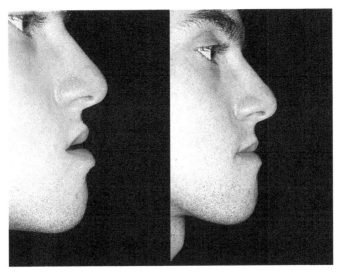

Figs. 7,8. Incompetent lips : contraction of the mentalis muscle during lip closure is evident

Particular attention should be paid to the relationship between lips and teeth and between lips and gingiva, both at rest and when smiling, considering tooth exposure and gummy smile, if any (Figure 9).

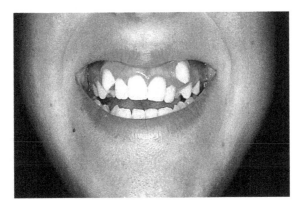

Fig. 9. Tipical gummy smile

Lastly, the nasolabial angle and the paranasal areas must be evaluated and examined for depressions as well as the naso-genial fold, which in some cases may be highly accentuated (Figure 10).
With regard to the clinical examination of the lower third of the face, the overall shape of the mandible should be evaluated, considering the characteristics and position of angles of the mandible, the shape and symmetry of the chin, the presence and extent of the labiomental fold; it is also important to evaluate the shape and characteristics of the angle between neck and chin and the soft tissues beneath the chin (thickness, tone, hypertrophy, excess of soft or adipose tissue) . The endoral examination must only in part be dedicated to the inter-arch relationship (Figure 11).

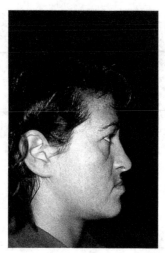

Fig. 10. Depression in paranasal areas

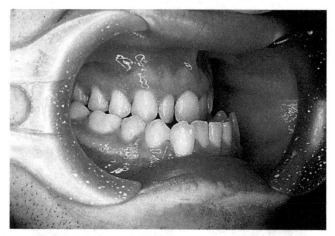

Fig. 11. Tipical example of class III malocclusion

In practice the most significant aspect in this connection consists in quantifying the negative over-jet evaluated at the incisal level; any anterior open bite should also be evaluated. Right from the first examination it is necessary to become used to seeing the two arches independently, since this is the way they will be treated and prepared for definitive surgical correction. The presence and number of teeth must be evaluated, any cases of agenesis, presence of tooth rotation, extent of crowding. The periodontal condition above all of the lower incisors must be carefully evaluated (Figure 12), these being the critical points in the treatment plan for these patients.

Simple clinical examination can reveal the presence and extent of dental compensation at this level. The quality and quantity of adherent gingiva must be evaluated, as must any pockets, the characteristics of the frenulum linguae and of the frenulum labii inferioris.

Lastly, true macroglossia (a very rare condition) must be determined, alongside the presence of undesirable habits and/or swallowing abnormalities.

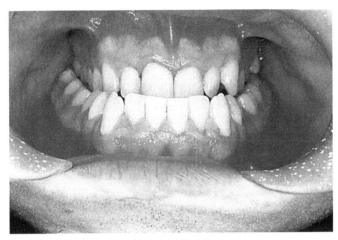

Fig. 12. Lower incisors and their periodontal evaluation

Radiological examination including full panoramic orthopantomography completes the clinical examination of the tooth arches, providing useful elements concerning the presence of any impacted teeth and on the inclination and direction of tooth roots.

3. Cephalometry

An enormous amount has been written on the question of cephalometric analysis in dentofacial anomalies, from Schwarz (1954) analysis of the profile to the more recent and sophisticated analyses by Arnett & Bergman (1993) , via intermediate contributions from Fish & Epker (1980) , and Ricketts (1961). In reality each of these analyses reflects its author's philosophy and intentions, privileging skeletal relationships or those of the soft tissues according to taste.

Cephalometric analysis on a radiograph taken in lateral projection is without doubt an excellent method to study the relationships between skeletal structures and between these and the soft tissues and teeth. It is useful for orthodontic planning of any extractions and consequent choice of anchorage, and it is also a useful tool to verify orthodontic treatment that has been performed in function of profilometric changes. Cephalometry must not however be used as the primary component in diagnosis.

The primary aim of treatment is not to bring cephalometric values within the normal range, but rather to make facial esthetics attractive and to allows a good chewing function, regarding muscular balance and tmj movements. Nevertheless, reaching these two goals is not extremely simple and easy to interpret.

In our opinion cephalometric analysis, in the sphere of orthodontic-surgical treatment, must be extremely simple and easy to interpret, both in the diagnostic phase and during treatment planning; it must also always and constantly be related and integrated with aesthetic clinical examination, and in the case of a discrepancy (always possible!) between the two evaluations, the one that is most useful to achieve our specific aesthetic or functional goal must be followed, on the merits of the individual case.

Cephalometric analysis includes angular and linear skeletal measurements, measurement of the relationship between bony bases and the base of the skull, measurement of soft tissues and/or aesthetic evaluations, dentobasal and dentoskeletal relationships, in all cases respecting the concepts of simplicity and pragmatism given above.

Lateral radiographs must be taken with the teeth in centric relation and the lips in the rest position. The centric relation is always used except in those cases in which there is a marked discrepancy between centric relation and habitual relation. In this case two radiographs are taken, one in centric relation and the other in the habitual position: on that taken in centric relation the sagittal relationship between maxilla and mandible is determined, whereas that taken in the habitual relation is used to measure the vertical dimensions.

In our analysis, the values are subdivided into five groups: maxilla, mandible, vertical parameters, dental parameters and soft tissues.

With regard to the bony bases, we take into consideration three angular measurements to evaluate their position three-dimensionally, and a linear anthropometric measurement to determine length and development. Evaluation of soft tissues, as also that of the vertical dimension, follows the indications given by Fish & Epker (1980) , in their turn taken from Ricketts (1961) analysis (Fig. 13, 14, 15, 16). Nevertheless, all strictly cephalometric and geometric considerations must always be integrated and compared with clinical and aesthetic considerations, and in the case of any discrepancy the surgeon's or the orthodontist's experience and intuition must, as the case merits, privilege clinical diagnosis or cephalometric analysis. Frequently, the final decision will be based on aesthetic considerations.

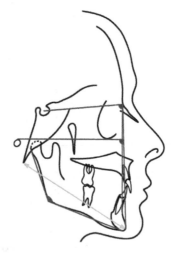

Fig. 13. Mandibular angular (red) and linear parameters (green)

For the mandible the reference values in cephalometric analysis consist of three angular and one linear measurement

The first angle is the angle SNB; the normal value is 80+-2° in men and 78+-2° in women. As in the case of the maxilla, this value is confirmed by the angle at which the Frankfurt plane meets the line N-Pog. The latter value is 89+-3°. These values enable us to determine the antero-posterior position of the mandible.

The linear distance measured from the line joining the basion and the pogonion provides further confirmation concerning size and position of the mandible.

The last measurement taken into consideration is the gonial angle. This value, normally in the range 130+-7°, gives useful indications both for evaluation of the sagittal position of the mandible and, when related to vertical parameters, in studying vertical anomalies and open bite.

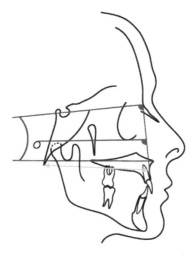

Fig. 14. Maxillary angular (red) and linear parameters (green)

The maxilla is analyzed in relation to the base of the skull in the sagittal and vertical sense by determining three angles and one linear measurement: the angle SNA, the angle Frankfurt/Na, the craniospinal angle, plus the length of the line Ba-A .

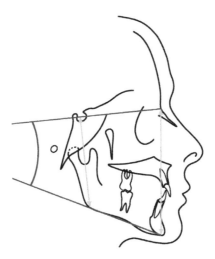

Fig. 15. Vertical angular (red) and linear parameters (green)

The angle SNA, whose normal value is in the range 82+-2° in men and 80+-2° in women, can be to some extent conditioned by the inclination of the plane SN, therefore another angular value is also taken into consideration, that at which the Frankfurt plane meets the line passing through NA. This latter value is normally 90+-3°. This value indicates the antero-posterior position of the maxilla and aids interpretation of dentoskeletal anomalies.

The craniospinal angle (that between the bispinal plane and the plane SN) indicates the position of the maxilla with regard to the base of the skull and may reveal any rotation of the maxilla clockwise or anti-clockwise; this evaluation is very important in diagnosing and planning treatment for open bite (normal value 10+-3°).

Lastly, the antero-posterior position of the maxilla and its sagittal development are confirmed by measuring the line Ba-A, that is the distance between the basion and point A. This value is normally 94+-6 mm in men and 88+-4 mm in women.

The vertical dimension, from the skeletal standpoint, is studied by measuring the angle between the mandible and the base of the skull and the relationship between anterior and posterior vertical dimensions. The angle Go-Me/SN is equal to 32+-4°; wider or narrower values of this angle objectively indicate the presence of open bite or deep bite.

The relationship between anterior and posterior vertical dimension is determined by measuring the segments S-Go and N-Me. This ratio is normally 62+-3%. This parameter enables us to establish with some accuracy whether the subject is normo-, hyper- or hypo-divergent.

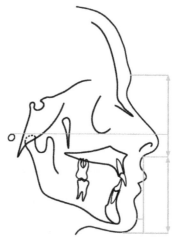

Fig. 16. Linear parameters (green) for the soft tissues

Different types of profilometric analysis have been proposed for the soft tissues . Figure 16 illustrates the analysis method we use, which is extrapolated from analyses by Fish & Epker (1980) and uses the perpendicular to the Frankfurt plane.

In the first instance we observe the ratio between the median third and the lower third, that is between the glabella-subnasale and subnasale-soft tissue menton distances. This ratio is normally 1:1.

We then measure the length of the upper lip, joining the subnasale to the stomion. The normal value is 22+-2 mm in men and 20+-2 mm mm in women; below these values the subject is said to have a short upper lip.

Another reference value in studying the soft tissues is the inter-labial distance. This is measured as the distance between the stomion of the upper lip and the stomion of the lower lip, obviously with the lips in the rest position. Normal values vary from 0 - 3 mm, although higher values are now also accepted, up to 5 mm . Values above 5 mm indicate incompetent lips.

There are also three values that indicate the antero-posterior position of the soft tissues, lips and chin. In this connection we measure the distance from the stomion of the upper and that of the lower lip to a straight line passing through the subnasale perpendicular to the Frankfurt plane. For the upper lip, normal values are between –2 and +2 mm; for the lower lip between –4 and 0 mm. The distance from the same line to the soft tissue pogonion indicates the position of the chin; normal values are between –6 and -2 mm. Naturally, all these numerical evaluations must be related to the overall aesthetics of the face.

On the contrary, where cephalometric analysis has an irreplaceable, almost a dogmatic, value is with regard to the position and inclination of the maxillary and mandibular incisors; their inclination with regard to their respective bony bases must always be rigorously sought and achieved: 109° to the bispinal plane for the maxillary incisors, and 90° to the mandibular plane (Go-Me) for the mandibular incisors.

In the case of significant rotational movements of the maxilla, inclination of the maxillary incisor to the S-N plane must also be taken into consideration; this situation comes about above all in cases of open bite. Compromise solutions over the position of the incisors with respect to their bone bases should only be contemplated where periodontal problems limit the possible orthodontic movement.

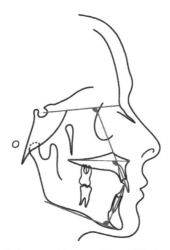

Fig. 17. Angular parameters (red) for maxillary and mandibular incisors

As we have already said, the study of dental relationships is undoubtedly the most important component of cephalometric analysis. These are the only values that, with rare exceptions, must always be brought within the normal range. The cephalometric analysis of the relationships between the incisors and their respective bony bases is the true guide for planning pre-surgical orthodontic treatment, and substantially is the fulcrum of orthodontic decompensation. These values also guide us in the need for any tooth extractions and the choice of anchorage.

As far as the maxillary incisors are concerned, the tooth axis normally forms an angle of 109+-5° with the bispinal plane, and this value must always be respected. The primary task of orthodontic treatment is to bring these values within the normal range. It is known that in cases of dentoskeletal anomaly, the teeth tend to move to compensate for the malocclusion, in an attempt to achieve contact. Thus it is almost normal to find an increased value of this angle in Class III subjects.

Another very important value is the angle the axis of the maxillary incisor forms with the cranial base. The normal value is 103+-2°, and this serves as a point of reference in cases of surgical rotation of the maxilla to correct open bite. In these cases, obviously the bispinal plane also changes, so that a comparison of the two values enables us to modulate the extent of movement of the maxillary incisors.

Another important value that may be considered in the spatial evaluation of the maxillary incisors is the distance between the perpendicular to the Frankfurt plane passing through point A and the most anterior point of the crown of the maxillary incisor. This value is 4 mm.

The same may be said for the mandibular incisor, whose axis forms an angle of 90+-5° with the mandibular base Go-Me. A decrease in this angle is almost always found in Class III subjects, as a compensatory factor for malocclusion.

These are the only cephalometric values that must almost always be normalized, hence the importance of orthodontic planning, because these values will guide us in sagittal movements and in the choice of any necessary extractions to achieve good orthodontic decompensation.

4. Pre-surgical orthodontic treatment

4.1 General principles

Pre-operative orthodontic treatment must aim to obtain two ideal arches capable of being coordinated, with each tooth in the correct position, always treating the two arches separately, and always bearing in mind the goals of the subsequent surgical repositioning.

In order to correctly approach pre-operative orthodontic treatment, careful study of the casts is fundamental. Initially they must be analyzed separately: the shape of the arch (parabolic, triangular, square), the extent of crowding, tooth rotation and the curve of Spee must be evaluated.

Only after this preliminary examination should the relationship between the two arches be examined. It is sufficient initially to position the casts manually with the molars in Class I occlusion, so as to evaluate discrepancies between the two arches that impede their co-ordination and to gain the first general indications concerning the requirements and goals of pre-operative orthodontic treatment (Figure 18). After this first brief and general indication, the first thing to be examined is the position of the maxillary and mandibular incisors, and any crowding. The entire orthodontic treatment plan will be developed from these evaluations as will be explained in detail successively.

With regard to the type of equipment and techniques to be used, we believe that standard equipment and the simplest and most widely used orthodontic techniques are preferable. Brackets cemented directly onto the teeth are perfectly acceptable even for orthodontic-surgical treatment.

Ceramic brackets may be used in the anterior maxillary sector, from canine to canine, whereas metallic attachments are always preferable in the mandibular arch.The first and second molars must always be banded.

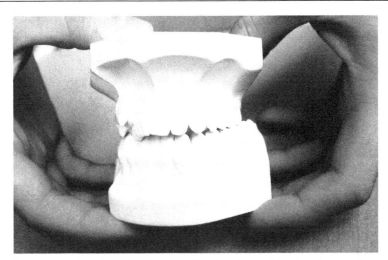

Fig. 18. Preliminary evaluation of arches coordination by positioning the casts in molars class I relationship (see 4.1 general principles)

With regard to the height at which to cement the brackets, on the mandibular arch they must be placed 0.5 - 1 mm more apically than normal to allow for intra-operative and immediate post-operative requirements.

The goals and basic concepts of orthodontic preparation may be subdivided thus: *position of incisors, transverse coordination, dental midlines, symmetry of canines, curve of Spee* (Ronchi, 2005). We will analyze each aspect separately.

4.2 Position of incisors

As we have already said, this is an essential point in all orthodontic-surgical treatment and should probably be considered one of its key points.

Restoration of the correct inclination of the incisors versus their respective bony bases thus becomes a condition "sine qua non" in pre-operative orthodontic treatment. Reference parameters for correct evaluation are exclusively of the cephalometric type. The most suitable and reliable cephalometric values are the inclination of the maxillary incisors on the bispinal plane and that of the mandibular incisors on the mandibular plane (generally Go-Men).

Restoration of the correct position of the incisors, also defined as decompensation, together with correction of any crowding, of necessity dictate whether or not tooth extractions will be required. Normally, mild to moderate crowding of the mandibular arch can be resolved through vestibularization of the incisors without requiring extraction. In general, crowding of 2-3 mm per hemiarch can be resolved in this way; in most cases, correction of the inclination of the incisors is achieved simply by using increasingly heavy square or rectangular archwires. Obviously, in calculating spaces to correct crowding, the starting position and the planned final position of the mandibular incisors must be taken into consideration. In more severe crowding, above 4 mm per hemiarch, the first or second premolars are extracted, depending on whether the crowding is more marked in the anterior or posterior arch sectors . In some situations, tooth condition (extensive carries, root-canal therapy) may dictate extractions.

Similar considerations apply to the maxillary incisors. Since in a high percentage of cases they are markedly vestibularized, decompensation at this level requires an amount of space that can often only be gained by extracting the first premolars. Whether or not therapeutic extraction of premolars is planned obviously conditions the final molar relationship: if extractions are limited to the maxillary arch the final molar relationship will be Class II; if no teeth are extracted, or if they are extracted from both arches, the final molar relationship will be Class I. Therapeutic extractions of the mandibular first premolars in Class III of necessity also involves extracting the maxillary first or second premolars.

The orthodontic procedures required to prepare these patients for surgery (extraction of upper teeth but frequently not of lower teeth, Class II elastics) are thus the exact opposite of corrective orthodontic treatment, and thus produce a temporary worsening of the situation. It is therefore essential to explain this temporary worsening of the functional and aesthetic situation to the patient.

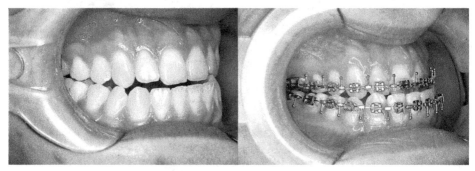

Figs. 19, 20. Decompensation of mandibular incisors

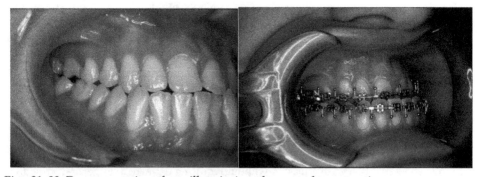

Figs. 21, 22. Decompensation of maxillary incisors by premolars extraction

4.3 Transverse coordination

With regard to this aspect, two fundamental concepts must be taken into account: how to evaluate any lack of transverse coordination, and how to correct it.

As we already said, right from the start of treatment we must become accustomed to looking at each arch independently, so that the transverse relationship must be evaluated on each plaster cast singly, and never on the endoral clinical examination. Furthermore, this step must only be done after having decided on any premolars destined for extraction, and thus after having established what the molar relationship will be at the end of treatment (molar Class I or Class II). At this point, simply by taking hold of the plaster casts and placing the molars in the planned final relationship, we have a clear view of the transverse relationship and of any need to correct it (Figure 20).

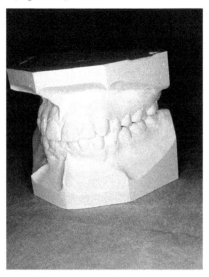

Fig. 23. Evaluating the casts in a Class I relationship shows an acceptable transverse coordination

In Class III an apparent contraction of the maxilla frequently resolves spontaneously simply through sagittal displacement of the bony bases.
In cases in which there is true contraction of the maxilla, the extent of the required expansion must be established, as well as deciding how it can best be achieved. A basic concept is to apply approximately 20% over-correction of the transverse defect; if the transverse deficiency, as measured on the plaster casts, is 3 mm, then orthodontic expansion should be 4 mm.

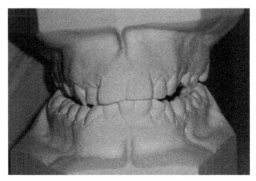

Fig. 24. Evaluating the casts in a Class I relationship shows a true narrowness of the maxillary arch

Even in a patient who has completed growth, expansion of up to 4 mm can generally be obtained orthodontically (through expansion arches, palato-vestibular torque in posterior sectors, Quad-Helix). For values above 4 mm, on the contrary, orthopedic approaches are necessary, such as disjunction of the palatine suture. This procedure may easily be performed in patients up to 16 years of age with the classic palatal torque expansion device cemented onto premolars and molars. Surgically-assisted expansion, which employs osteotomy lines similar to those of the Le Fort I osteotomy, is always necessary above the age of 18 years. In patients between the ages of 16 and 18, the choice of orthopedic or surgically-assisted expansion must take into consideration the patient's skeletal structure (subjects with large bones and with clinical or radiographic signs that growth is complete); in some cases, evaluation of the carpal index; the radiographic appearance of the suture; in any case, for expansions above 8 mm; lastly, cases of failed purely orthopedic expansion.

Once expansion has been achieved, the expansion device must be kept in place for approximately four months. Fixed appliance therapy must follow immediately: the two steps must always take place in a single appointment to avoid the risk of early relapse.

In general, if rapid palatal expansion is required, it should be the first procedure of the entire pre-operative treatment.

4.4 Dental midlines
The concept that must guide the orthodontist and surgeon through all planning and operative phases is that, once treatment is completed, the two dental midlines must coincide not only with one another, but must of necessity fall on the facial midline axis. By "facial midline axis" we mean the axis drawn perpendicular to the bipupillar line, in cases of clinical evaluation, or the axis drawn perpendicular to the line that joins the fronto-zygomatic suture, in the case of postero-anterior cephalometric evaluation. Furthermore, the point that characterizes the mental symphysis must also coincide with the facial midline axis. A discrepancy of 1 mm between the two dental midlines and the facial midline axis may be tolerated

Thus, the ideal and theoretical goal of all pre-operative orthodontic treatment is that the maxillary dental midline coincide with the facial midline axis and that the mandibular dental midline must coincide with the line of mental symphysis; unfortunately, in some cases insuperable orthodontic limits make this impossible.

Concerning the maxilla, initial deviation of the dental midline above 3 mm, requires in general surgical repositioning of the maxilla; the same, in the mandible, when the initial deviation of dental midline is more than 3 mm from symphyisis line, a compensatory genioplasty with lateral translation must be planned.

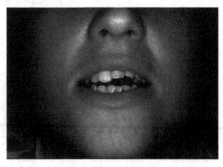

Fig. 25. Evident deviation of the maxillary dental midline with regard to tha facial axis

In case where maxillary osteotomy alone is planned, it is mandatory that orthodontic preparation of mandibular arch perfectly center mandibular dental midline to the facial axis; and the same, when mandibular osteotomy alone is planned, it is necessary that maxillary dental midline exactly coincide with the facial axis. In case when bimaxillary osteotomy is planned, the superimposition of dental midlines and facial axis will be achieved surgically.

4.5 Symmetry of canines
The position of the canines constitutes another key point in pre-operative orthodontic treatment. It is imperative that these teeth occupy a symmetrical position in the two arches. Indeed, an asymmetrical position of the canines would inevitably cause lateral deviation or some form of dentofacial asymmetry.
Thus symmetry of the canines must be obtained through suitable mesio-distal or disto-mesial orthodontic tooth movement. In cases of accentuated asymmetry, strategic unilateral extraction of the premolars may be necessary to achieve this goal correctly.

4.6 Curve of spee
Analysis and management of the curve of Spee in pre-operative orthodontic treatment is of particular strategic importance. First of all it must be remembered that in Class III cases with mandibular dental compensation and tendency to covered bite there is often an accentuated mandibular curve of Spee. The decompensation of the mandibular incisors and leveling of the corresponding tooth arch automatically bring about a flattening of this curve; nevertheless the flattening must not be complete and some curvature, which we could define as physiological, must be maintained in order to simplify management of occlusion immediately post-surgery. Maintenance of some curvature of the mandibular arch enables post-surgical occlusion to be obtained with a slight over-bite (2-3 mm) that facilitates immediate post-surgery physiotherapy and helps to control any tendency to relapse in subsequent weeks and months.
The maintenance of curve of Spee on the inferior arch, associated with an anterior over-bite, necessarily implies, as an inevitable corollary, that the position of the brackets on the mandibular teeth must be 0.5-1 mm more apical than normal positions used in orthodontics, at the least from the first premolars forwards.

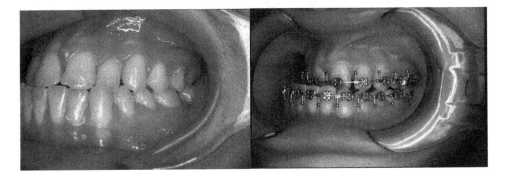

Figs. 26,27. Correction of curve of Spee

In patients with associated anterior open bite, maintaining or increasing curve of Spee must be further exasperated to obtain an over-bite of 3 mm. The position of the mandibular brackets must also be adequate for this purpose. Furthermore, the curvature of the maxillary arch must be maintained and perfectly adapted to the mandibular arch, carefully avoiding creating any posterior lateral open bite, which would bring a high risk of post-operative relapse. Frequently, in patients with anterior open bite, the mandibular curve of Spee is initially flat or even inverse, and pre-operative orthodontic treatment must of necessity recreate a "physiological" curve of Spee.

4.7 New aesthetic appliances

New invisible appliances, like lingual tecnique and Invisilign, propagate in orthodontic field in the last years, to get a better compliance and satisfaction out of patients.

Lingual technique may involve some difficulties in pre-surgical treatment, during models analysis, because, in particular in superior arch, brackets could interfere with a correct occlusion and cause precontacts with the inferior arch.

Furthermore, in any case, during surgical and post-surgical phases vestibular appliances are necessary to make an intermaxillary temporary fixation or to positioning post-surgical occlusal elastic guide. Since a kind of appliance both vestibular and lingual is not thinkable, replace lingual tecnique with vestibular one, or prepare a vestibular device easily compatible with the lingual one, become unavoidable. Indeed, bars, in this case, are hardly to position and to manage.

In the following pictures we show an illustrative case.

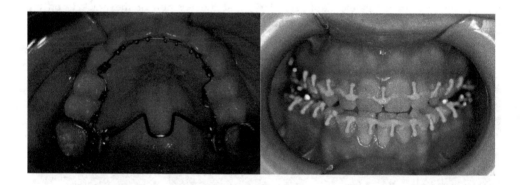

Figs. 28, 29. Example of lingual tecnhique

Invisilign treatment has certainly less difficulty, but dental movements with this technique may be limited, especially regarding extrusion, rotation and torque of the teeth. So, this kind of device is indicated in selected cases, and is it often necessary to change the technique into the traditional full-brackets vestibular appliance in the last phases of the presurgical orthodontic treatment.

However, if we want to make use of this tecnique for all the treatment length, and if that is possible from the orthodontic point of view, we have to use bars during surgical and immediatly post-surgical phases and, most important, a perfect surgical occlusion, without precontacts, is mandatory, because elastic occlusal guide has more effect on bars than on dental arches.

In the following pictures we show an illustrative case.

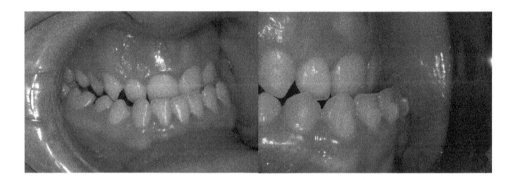

Figs. 30, 31. Full preoperative orthodontic treatment with Invisalign

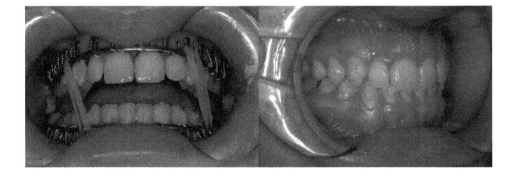

Figs. 32, 33. Immediate post-surgical phase with bars, and final occlusal result

5. Surgical procedure selection

Furthermore, surgical correction of Class III cases must always be postponed until growth is completed and thus, in general terms, not before 18 years of age for women and 19 or 20 for men. Surgical correction that is done too early can easily lead to a relapse due to residual mandibular growth.

The choice of surgical procedure to correct Class III cases essentially takes into account aesthetic evaluation in the three planes of space: sagittal, vertical, and transverse. It must answer the following question: which is more appropriate, a maxillary osteotomy, a mandibular osteotomy or a double jaw operation? Cephalometric analysis of skeletal structures takes second place after aesthetic considerations; if skeletal values are in agreement with the surgical approach selected on aesthetic grounds, so much the better; if not, then aesthetic evaluation should always dominate.

From the sagittal standpoint, the parameters that indicate advancement of the maxilla with Le Fort I osteotomy are: flattening of the paranasal areas, accentuated naso-genial fold, moderate flattening of the cheek-bones, obtuse nasolabial angle, maxillary prolabium little in evidence, prominent nose with some degree of hump and tip tilted downwards

Where a larger increase at the middle third is necessary, Bell's high osteotomy may be taken into consideration, because this provides greater filling at the cheek-bones (Bell et al, 1988)

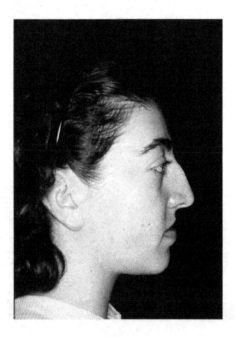

Fig. 34. Tipical case in wich is indicated an advancement Le Fort I ostetomy

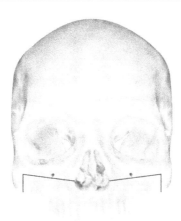

Fig. 35. High Le Fort I osteotomy according by Bell

In cases of severe hypoplasia of the middle third of the face, with flattening of the inferior orbital rim and scleral exposure, a maxillo-malar osteotomy may be employed (Keller & Sather 1987). However, this type of osteotomy only affords limited vertical or transverse movement and thus indications are specific: anomaly that is solely antero-posterior, normal or decreased vertical dimension, maxillary dental midline coinciding with the median axis of symmetry or at most deviated by 2 mm. In other cases, where this type of osteotomy cannot be adopted, the best alternative is the classic Le Fort I osteotomy associated with implantation of alloplastic material or lipofilling in the sub-orbital area.

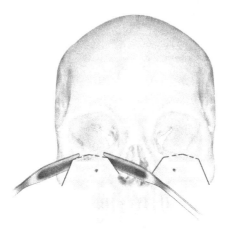

Fig. 36. Intraoral maxillo-malar osteotomy

In few selected cases, a true anterior position of the mandible and chin requires a mandibular set back alone. In this case it is necessary that cheek, nose and superior lip have a good balance. However, correction of Class III cases with mandibular osteotomy alone should be limited to clinical situations with negative over-jet not above 3-4 mm.

Indeed, marked mandibular setback may produce excess soft tissue beneath the chin, which is negative from the aesthetic standpoint, and cause a reduction of posterior airway space, with possible tendency to develop an OSAS in the future (Riley et al, 1987).

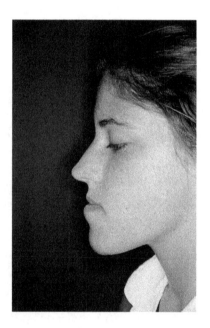

Fig. 37. Tipical case in wich is indicated a mandibular set back alone

In a great number of patients, for larger amount of initial over-jet, double jaw osteotomy should otherwise be preferred because it guarantees in these cases greater skeletal and muscular stability, a less stretching of the pterygomasseteric sling, and in order to avoid excessive bi-protrusion.

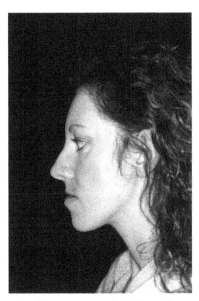

Fig. 38. Tipical case in wich a double osteotomy is indicated

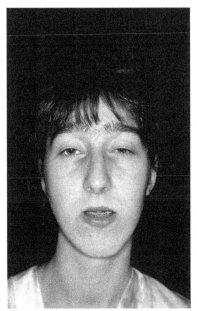

Fig. 39. Tipical case in wich is indicated a bimaxillary osteotomy with superior repositioning of the maxilla

With regard to the vertical dimension, the fundamental parameters to take into consideration are: relationship between lips and teeth, gummy smile if present, labial competence or incompetence, and the ratio between middle and lower thirds of the face. A vertical excess of the maxilla with labial incompetence, gummy smile and excessive tooth exposure tends to indicate repositioning the maxilla superiorly.

On the contrary, in a small percentage of cases characterized by little vertical development and insufficient tooth exposure (short face) repositioning the maxilla downward is indicated. If, on the contrary, the vertical excess is exclusively in the lower third, genioplasty with vertical reduction will be required.

With regard to transverse dimensions, these concern both the occlusal relationship and aesthetic parameters. From the occlusal standpoint, transverse discrepancy should be corrected, as we have already seen, during pre-operative orthodontic treatment. Only in some particular cases may segmental maxillary osteotomy, in two or more pieces, be taken into consideration. However, the transverse changes that can be obtained with these types of osteotomy are fairly limited: 4 – 5 mm with regard to maxillary expansion and this limitation is due to the fact that the palatine fibro-mucosa is not elastic (Proffit et al, 1996). With regard to aesthetics, the fundamental parameter in the transverse dimension is the ratio between the bi-zygomatic and the bi-gonial widths. In Class III cases there is usually a reduced bi-zygomatic width, and various methods exist to achieve an increase in this measurement, as lipofilling or biomaterial implants.

With regard to correction of the mandibular angles, this may quite easily be done endorally by remodeling with a pear-shaped bur, or through otsteotomy and resection with an angled saw.

6. Post-operative orthodontic treatment

In the first post-operative weeks, the active and passive physiotherapy is essential: active mandibular movements, again guided by elastics, are gradually increased. Normally, over a 2-week period, the patients achieve a substantial degree of mandibular opening, about 3.0 to 3.5 mm, and the physiotherapy is complete at about 4 to 6 weeks.

After the physiotherapy phase is finished, the patient may begin the final orthodontic treatment. The goal is to achieve occlusal relationships that we might define as ideal, in terms of canine class, molar class and coincidence of the dental midlines. In practice, in this phase some simple orthodontic maneuvers will suffice, such as closing any small residual diastemas, correcting a slight lateral cross-bite, perfecting intercuspidation, optimizing over-jet and over-bite.

Obviously the duration of the final orthodontic phase depends on the degree of preparation achieved during pre-surgical treatment. In most cases, however, two or three months will suffice.

Retention, in orthodontic-surgical treatment, serves the dual purpose of stabilizing tooth relationships and contributing to skeletal stability, although in our opinion this latter point depends to a greater extent on other factors, such as correct condylar position and condition of the musculature. It is, however, important to stress that good dental retention contributes to maintaining the final occlusion that was achieved surgically, guaranteeing occlusal stability, which will surely have positive repercussions on the final stability in the widest sense. In general, the methods used for retention are those used in traditional orthodontics rather than in surgical treatment.

Fixed retainers are normally preferred, applied to the mandibular and maxillary anterior sectors, in cases of high risk of dental relapse in these areas (resolution of tooth crowding without extraction, decompensation). In some cases, especially at the maxillary arch, it may be indicated to use removable retention plates of various types, for example to be worn at night, partly to guarantee stability of orthodontically and orthopedically corrected transverse relations.

7. Clinical cases

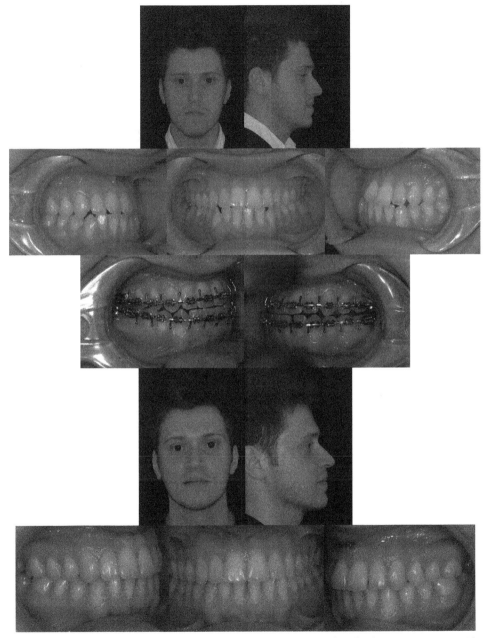

Case 1. Class III deformity with maxilla hypoplasia. Presurgical orthodontic treatment with Invisalign and vestibular brackets just on surgical phases. Surgical correction with Le Fort I maxillary osteotomy. Result two years later.

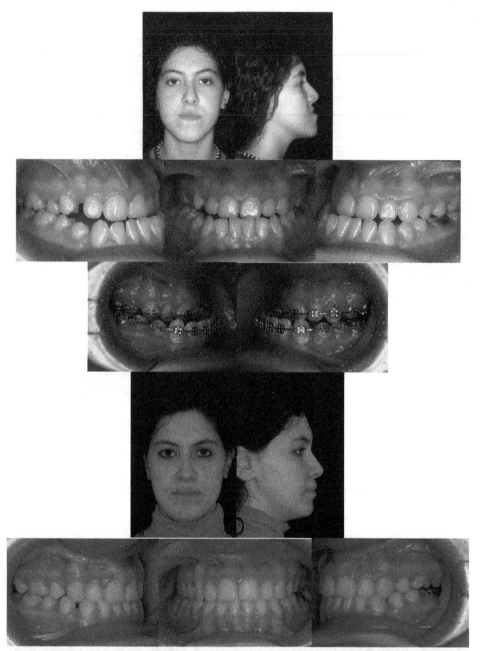

Case 2. Class III deformity. Presurgical orthodontic treatment with fixed appliance and decompensation of superior and inferior incisors, extraction of 14 and 24. Surgical correction with bimaxillary osteotomy (Le Fort I maxillary osteotomy and mandibular set back.) Result six years later

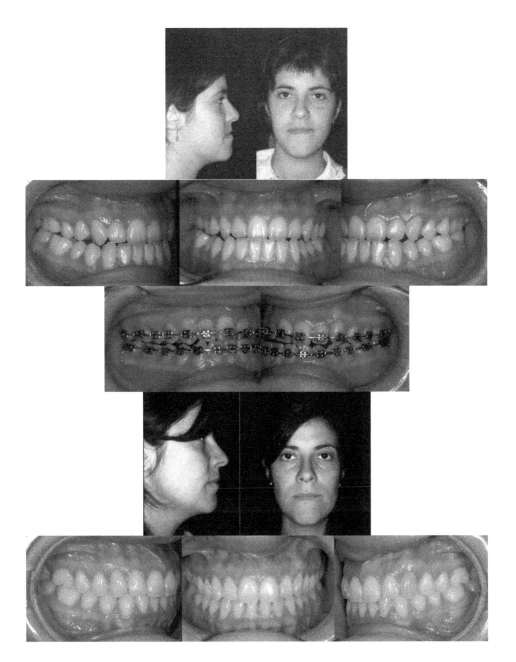

Case 3. Class III deformity. Presurgical orthodontic treatment with fixed appliance and decompensation of mandibular incisors. Surgical correction with mandibular set back alone. Result ten years later.

8. References

Arnett G.W., Bergman R.T. (1993) : Facial keys to orthodontic diagnosis and treatment planning. Part I *Am. J. Orthod. Dentofac. Orthop.* Vol. 103, pp. 299-312

Bell W.H., Mannai C., Luhr H.G. (1988) : Art and science of the Le Fort I downfracture. *Int.J.Adult. Orthod. Orthognath.Surg.* vol. 1, pp. 23-52

Fish L.C., Epker B.N. (1980) : Surgical-orthodontic cephalometric prediction tracing *J. Clin. Ortod.* vol. 14, pp. 36-52

Keller E.E., Sather A.H.   (1987): Intraoral quadrangular Le Fort II osteotomy. *J.Oral. Maxillofac. Surg.* Vol. 45, pp. 223-232

Laskin B.M., Ryan W.A., Greene C.S. (1986) : Incidence of temporomandibular symptoms in patients with major skeletal malocclusions: a survey of oral and maxillofacial surgery training programs *Oral. Surg. Oral. Med. Pathol.* vol. 61, pp. 537-541

Proffit W.R., Turvey T.A., Phillips C. (1996) : Orthognathic surgery : A hierarchy of stability *Int J Adult. Orthod. Orthognath. Surg.* vol. 11, pp.191-204.

Ricketts R.M. (1961) : Cephalometric analysis and synthesis *Angle Orthont.* vol. 31, pp. 141-156

Riley R.W., Powell N.B., Guilleminault C., Ware W. (1987) : Obstructive sleep apnea syndrome following surgery for mandibular prognathism. *J. Oral Maxillofac. Surg.* vol. 45, pp. 450-452

Ronchi P. : (2005) : *Orthodontic Surgical Treatment of Dentofacial Anomalies. An Integrated Estthetic Functional Approach.* Ed. Quintessence Publishing, ISNB 9708-0-86715-397, New Malden

Schwarz A.M. (1954) : Ueber eckzahnverlagerung und ihre Behebung *Fortchr-Kieferorthop* vol. 15, pp. 119-112

White C.S., Dolwick F. (1992) : Prevalence and variance of temporomandibular disfunction in orthognathic surgery patients. *Int.J. Adult. Orthod. Orthognath Surg* vol. 7, pp. 7-14

Part 2

Research

5

Does Comtemporary Orthodontics Comply with Universal Logic?

Hicham Khayat

Maitrise Universitaire en Orthodontie et Orthopédie Dento-Faciale
Diplôme Universitaire de Prothèse et de Réhabilitation Maxillo-Faciale
Diplôme Universitaire d'Implantologie Chirurgicale Orale et Maxillo-Faciale
Certificat post-universitaire de Radiologie Tridimensionnelle Dento-Maxillo-Faciale
Head of Polyclinique Dentaire Casablanca's Global care department
Morocco

1. Introduction

Contemporary orthodontic practice is segmented into schools and methods. These divisions within the specialty lay bare the lack of consensus on such fundamental issues as the conduct of the diagnosis, the design of a treatment plan or the fundamentals of appliance's mechanics! Such a situation would not be acceptable in any other medical discipline. Our purpose is to highlight a few inconsistencies responsible for this situation, under the harsh lights of philosophy and history of medicine.

2. Clinic

In the late eighteenth century, a new concept of Mankind takes place. Along with the development of sciences, the growing accumulation of knowledge boosted by the advances in printing, and an improved flow of knowledge. By grouping the patients in the same place-the hospital, initially a "mourroir"[1], a place where sicks were taken to die, the society, aiming to prevent epidemics, has extracted the patients from their own personal conditions, their homes and their family care; Thus Reducing the variability of forms of the same "disease" mainly related to the terrain; Thus making possible the observation of similarities in different patients. And finally society has created the conditions giving rise to another view, another thought: A new method based on the observation of symptoms and signs, the methodical and comprehensive grouping and consolidation of these "clinical signs"in "tables". This method took place although no one claimed to have built it and deeply contrasted with the previous discurses. The clinical method, that is to say modern medicine was born. It is constituted as a way of thinking opposed to the archaic medical practice. By "Clinique", was meant a "rationalist methodology" of medicine.

This original meaning has been forgotten over time. Many doctors today confuse it with office. This confusion may reflect the fact that in his genealogy, the clinic combines the knowledge, the Sick and the Institutions. As Michel Foucault has shown, its foundations are local, political and institutional factors. When the fundamentals changes, knowledge changes and sometimes loses. The doctors have forgotten the meaning of the Clinic. They have forgotten his former discoveries. Worse, doctors have forgotten that they have forgotten, willing to remember no more than the incompressible know-how mandatory to exercise: the technique.

As the clinic was established to accommodate the new, it disintegrates as it is no more than preserving what is already known, a repetition of what is already certain. Moreover, today, among the fundamental basis of contemporary orthodontics, medical marketing in all its forms, plays an increasingly important role.

Any theory always vanishes at the patient's bedside. The first premise of the clinical method is the perfect match between the visible and the expressible. Recovery without rest between the visible and the expressible. This is the logic of Condillac, the vision of a talking eye. With the clinical method, the eye finally cleared of chimeras is ready to welcome the new. And to describe it. Appoint to recognize. Recognize to treat. Probabilistic reasoning will appear and anatomopathology will assign a seat to evil in the very thickness of the living. But the Clinic which is whole based on this unprecedented relationship between vision and language should not be reduced to the systematic collection of signs already described. The "look" of the clinician, in any discipline is, and has to be the basis of any progress. Based on what is known as certain, with an extensive multi-disciplinary vocabulary, the true clinician will find the key point without losing his way gazing to everything and measuring everything. The eye must keep its edge. Beware of habits and systems. Reject the blinders of theory. Stay acute in order to detect the different, the new and the subtle.

3. Care givers and the principle of rationality

In preclinical times, men and women took over the health of their community, claiming to enjoy a mythical rationality[2]. The witch healers from prehistoric times invoked the devil. The priests of ancient times interceded for the patient with the divine (Serapis in Egypt, Apollo and Aesculapius in Greece ...). But the church abhorred blood: *Ecclesia abhorret a sanguine*. The monks of the Middle Ages are striving to console the sick: Question: Why does God allow us to endure such terrible evils? Answer: Because it is expedient for His glory and for the good of our soul. God is purifying its elected. He is not a judge who punishes. He is a father who corrects and chastises his beloved sons. And thus, the evils become great assets.The doctors were, mostly, members of the clergy and therefore unable to practice surgery. Surgery is thereby relegated to a lower rank in society, mainly performed by tooth-pullers, fairground merchants or barbers. They will become our ancestors, the "barber-surgeons", after a long conflict with the organized, educated and Latin-speaking body of physicians. With the clinical method and the more predictable and reproducible therapeutic results it provides, the care giver becomes a scientist. Accused yesterday of *mentir comme un arracheur de dents* (NDLT: "lying like a tooth-puller") dentists today aspires to an evidence-based practice.

Contemporary Orthodontics is a living example of the decline of the clinic. For many renowned authors, performing a diagnostic is no more than obtaining senseless measures compared to meaningless tables the only justification for which being the fact that everyone uses them. It rejects the individual in a face or a smile, while the clinic was established to the contrary from the individual, to welcome the new far from any dogmatic closure.

Treatments are standardized. As the barber who only deals with bleeding, we simply perform the same techniques reported by few measures and a programmable frame of mind, moving away from the path of Hippocrates who was attached to the observation and despised any form of system.You have to observe and to look askew. As mentioned by

Michel Foucault, "Looking askew" is a productive intellectual tactic, a must for clinical way of thinking. This is an invitation to observe from a novel standpoint, the intellectual processes by which we assess the functional or aesthetic situation of our patients and transform it into a good outcome through our diagnosis and our treatment.

4. Seeing, knowing, treating

Looking askew is the condition of birth of new thinking and relevant mind processes. Learning to see better, to see differently, learning to describe better. This is the only approach that always has and can still allow the emergence of better paradigms in phase with the up-to-date knowledge and cutting-edge technologies. See the subject but also its further investigations. Open to all vocabularies of modern dentistry and more broadly to any exact and universal knowledge.

5. Measuring, calculating, executing

In contrario, the "ready to wear thought system", and its inconsistencies, violate the fundamental clinical postulate, veiled the eyes of the practitioner, format his vocabulary and confine his arguments. The technique comfortably installs the practitioner in a robot status from witch that may be difficult to break free. Retreating into its certainties, abdicating critical sens and without curiosity about the fundamentals, the practitioner takes the risk of falling into dogmatism. The speech, the challenges and promises of the Clinic are threatened with extinction in the furrows of the technique and repetition.Today, orthodontic diagnosis is often based on a "fetishist" methodology : The dimensional statistical cephalometry.
Implicitly, this assumes that there is a cephalometrical numerical standard, a geometric "ideal" [3]canvas which can serve as an *étalon* to establish a diagnosis, develop a treatment plan and express a prognosis. This contradicts the morphological and biological variability of living organisms. The majority of cephalometric analysis authors has cautioned against the misuse of their own indicators and have sometimes confessed to their arbitrary. Nevertheless, the ease of the method, compatible with delegation and mass-practice orthodontics has assured its wide spreading among doctors and scholars. In the other hand, a relevant vision of the human head brought by architectural analysis does exists. Here, the clinician's eye look at the pillars, beams, arches and voids that form a functional structure, lively and full of meaning: The scene and spectacle of oral and facial function.
Once and for all, our purpose is not to condemn cephalometry. It keeps sens as a comparative or statistical tool, but to warn against shortcuts ang this kind of magic thinking that transforms a few integers without any clinical signification into a diagnostic panacea. Warn against The Mismeasure of Man. Againt this "eugenic" Violence of caregivers, forcing life-wide "cases" into narrow "boxes".The difference is enormous between a physician who takes the time to observe and one who "reads" labels, pasted on a radiological shadow.The aesthetics, which occupies a central place in the pattern of consultation and the therapeutic purpose is rarely the subject of academic teaching in our specialty. Straight lines, disastrous shortcuts of hurry thinking[4], hides the faces. Blind clinician Eyes.

6. Recipes instead of thinking

We see the tooth moving but, in reality,it is the socket that moves. Mechanics is the essence of orthodontic treatment. The resulting forces at the periodontal interface multiplied by the amount of tooth displacement is a mechanical energy than is expressed in joules. Thus, for an equal outcome, the best treatment, the most respectful, may well be that which minimizes the total energy transmitted to the periodontal tissues, labile but delicate. Periodontium, as a biological entity, is blind to the endless sophistications of our self-ligating or heat-memory fireworks. Only count the pressures that stimulate or otherwise degrade it. Primum non nocere.Basically, a force is an active ingredient, similar to a pharmacological molecule. The analogy is fruitful since the application point and direction of a force, as the tropism of a molecule, determines the target tissue. The intensity of a force equals to the dosimetry and the duration of exposure to the setting time. In the state of the art, and unusually for orthodontics, we accept that overdosing, over-treatment or bad prescription are not the key poiny.The debate focuses mainly on "ideal" bracket "information", easy opening, easy closing, etcetera. Magic thinking again. Marketing as the foundation of the clinic.Mechanics is an exact science, fortunately, as every day our lives depends on it. Nevertheless, it is never treated seriously. The vast majority of orthodontic literature figures are senseless from a "mechanical" point of view. Several authors have based upon physicists mechanics and contributed to the successful rationalization of orthodontic's mechanics. Their universal input does not enjoy the same penetration in the professional body that the ready to wear technique. They offen have nothing to sale and therefore no communication budget !

Sapere aude! Dare to think, "cried Emmanuel Kant to his contemporaries to help them break free of the intellectual minority[5]. The field of the unthought in orthodontics is much wider than one might think at first sight. The advent of evidence-based orthodontics in the soil of fetishism and inconsistencies of the specialty is problematic. A cure of common sense is highly indicated . "Common sense is the best shared thing in the world, for everyone thinks he is so well equipped that even those who are hardest to satisfy in everything else do not usually want to have more than they do. And as the diversity of our opinions do not come from what some are more reasonable than others, but only that we conduct our thoughts in various ways, and do not consider the same things "[6]

7. Conclusion

Turning his back on exact sciences and universal knowledge, the contemporary orthodontic practice is locked into normalized and similar techniques. Major Clinical issues are sinking in the furrows of repetition. In this context, the research is often a daily checking of what is already known. Innovations are too often minor improvements of what is already used. It will be interesting to retrieve all the subversive potential of the true Clinical method. Subversive in the truest sense, which is put in reverse, move things, violate the order things establish between themselves, and finally overcome them. It is urgent to move away from dogmatic closure. There hides the promises of the clinic.

8. References

[1] Foucault M, Naissance de la Clinique] XXXX
[2] Lebrun S] Se soigner autrefois] Médecins, saints et sorciers au XVII° et XVIII° siècles] Histoire.
[3] Gould S.J] The Mismeasure of Man] New York] WW Norton.
[4] Sabot P] L'Expérience, le savoir et l'Histoire dans les premiers écrits de Michel Foucault] Archives de Philosophie 2006 ;69 :285-303.
[5] Kant I] Was ist Aufklarung ? Berlinische Monatschrifte, 1784.
[6] Desccartes R] Le discours de la méthode] 1637.

Biomechanics of Tooth-Movement: Current Look at Orthodontic Fundamental

Joanna Antoszewska[1] and Nazan Küçükkeleş[2]
[1]*Wroclaw Medical University,*
[2]*Marmara University,*
[1]*Poland*
[2]*Turkey*

1. Introduction

Numerous methods of efficient orthodontic tooth-movement have been described in the literature for over 100 years, since Edward Hartley Angle had introduced foundations of malocclusion treatment (fig. 1). In such long term, different treatment philosophies have been permanently encountering beginning from Tweed[1] and his extraction concept versus

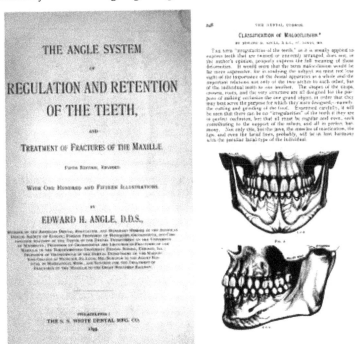

Fig. 1. Beginning of former century: philosophy proposed by the father of Orthodontic School, E.H. Angle

orthopedic functional expansion approach of acknowledged masters, such as: Andresen, Bimler, Klammt, Fränkel, Stockfish or Balters[2] (fig. 2a, b). Numerous appliances and techniques have been designed to accomplish treatment goals assumed by advocates and followers of both schools, especially challenging in adults who more and more frequently seek orthodontic care. Evidence based efficiency of sliding mechanics[3] and segmented technique[4-11] mostly related to the space closure (fig. 3a-c), maxillary enlargement in different skeletal configurations: class III[12-25] or II[26-28] prior to mandibular advancement or distalization of maxilla[29-46] are approaches of choice in non-extraction protocol.

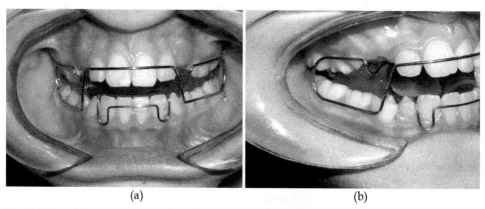

| (a) | (b) |

Fig. 2. Balters' bionator in situ: a) en face view, b) right side

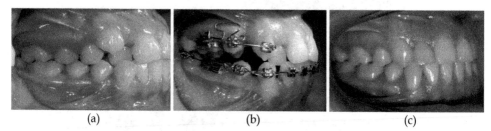

| (a) | (b) | (c) |

Fig. 3. Space closure with T-loop segmented archwire: a) initial occlusion, right side, b) T-loop in situ, c) final occlusion, right side

Independently on the treatment plan calling either for reduction of teeth number or dental arch expansion and despite modern and sophisticated orthodontic appliance or technique, even the most currently performed dental movements base on Newton's 3rd law established already in 1687: *to every action there is always opposed an equal reaction or the mutual actions of two bodies upon each other are always equal, and directed to contrary parts*[47]. Such fundamental enlightened orthodontist - beyond the shadow of the doubt - that any teeth-anchored desired movement produced the undesired one and the latter was to be carefully predicted thus fully controlled (fig. 4a, b). Meticulous evaluation of moments and forces resulting from planned tooth displacement[48-51], unavoidable for "orthodontic-driven" and efficient tooth-movement, initiated development of biomechanics: pure physics transferred into the oral cavity (fig. 5a-c, 6a-c). The concept resulted in deliberate anchorage reinforcement: increase of resistance of fulcrum located either in on teeth or skeletal structures[52].

Anchorage may be reinforced utilizing: a) extra-oral skeletal structures, b) teeth and intra-oral skeletal structures.

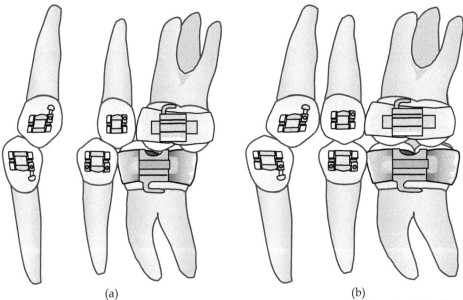

(a)   (b)

Fig. 4. Anchorage loss during canine retraction: a) initially - class I on both sides b) finally – cusp to cusp relationship due to mesial displacement of upper molars

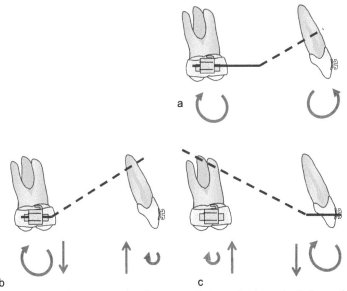

Fig. 5. Force vectors and moments displacing teeth in sagittal-vertical plane, depending on localization of the archwire bending between canine and 1st molar (provided there are no brackets on premolars): a) middle of the distance, b) close to 1st molar, c) close to a canine

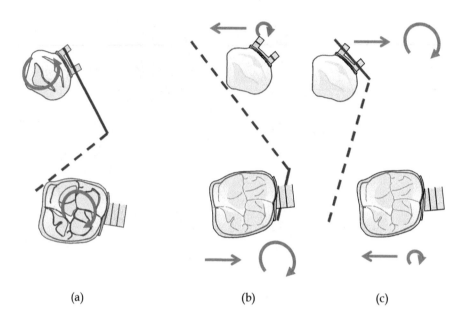

Fig. 6. Force vectors and moments displacing teeth in occlusal plane, depending on localization of the archwire bending between canine and 1st molar (provided there are no brackets on premolars): a) middle of the distance, b) close to 1st molar, c) close to a canine

a. Extra-oral appliances

Headgear - known already in 19th century allows orthodontic reacting forces pass through cranium and back bone: immobile structures, thus absolute anchorage is achieved. Position of external arms of the face bow dictates line force, in other words: enable precise prediction of the desired direction of tooth-movement[53] (fig. 7a-c). In order to adjust the line force, molar center of resistance must be established first. According to Schmuth et al.[54] such location may be easily predicted in several steps: 1) the face-bow, after adjustment of internal arms must lie flat on the surface, 2) reference points must be marked on external arms, 3 mm mesially to the ends of internal ones, 3) once the face-bow has been inserted in to the headgear tubes, next reference points must be marked 8 mm above the previous ones, on the patient's skin (fig. 8). Precisely designed headgear (fig. 9a-c) is mainly applied for correction of class II; nevertheless it may also be used for correction of class I with crowding in both jaws, in combination with fixed mechanics (fig. 10).

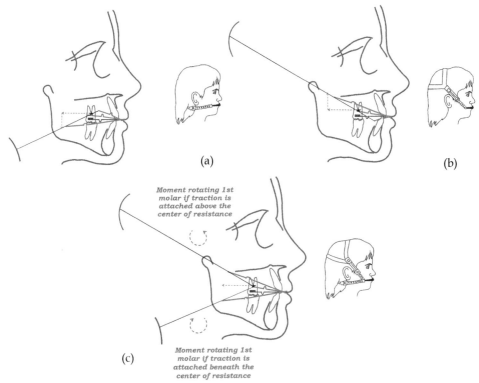

(a)

(b)

Moment rotating 1st
molar if traction is
attached above the
center of resistance

(c)

Moment rotating 1st
molar if traction is
attached beneath the
center of resistance

Fig. 7. Headgear - force vectors depending on position of external traction: a) low-pull, b) high-pull ; c) combi-pull; note that elimination of molar rotating moments depends on either the length as well as on angulation of face bow external arms

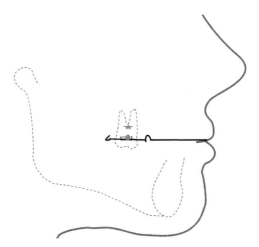

Fig. 8. Headgear adjustment: marking the center of molar resistance (asterisk) on patient's skin

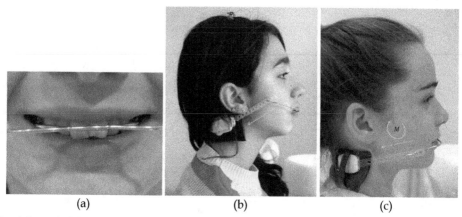

(a)   (b)   (c)

Fig. 9. Low pull headgear adjusted for class II treatment: a) en face view: position of face bow: it does not lean against lips, b) lateral view - external arms of the face bow bent up, c) external arms of the face bow bent down; note the direction of force line (———➤) and moment (M) rotating molar.

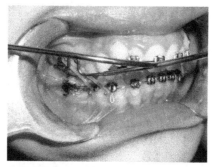

Fig. 10. Headgear combined with fixed appliances: intermaxillary class III traction forces lower canine distally

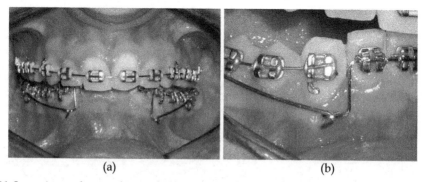

(a)   (b)

Fig. 11. Intrusion arch according to Burstone a) en face, in situ, b) connection of cantilever with front segment

Current mathematic calculations of forces couneracting reactive ones resulting from the front teeth movement are presented by Braun[55]. Burstone's intrusion arch (fig. 11a, b) while intruding upper incisors with the 50 g of force, simultaneously extrudes molars with the same force value. To prevent the latter phenomenon, high-pull headgear is to be worn 8 hours per day. It is illustrated with the formula: F_1 x 8h = 50 g x 24h, where F_1 = 150 g is a vertical component of the force produced by high-pull traction (fig. 12). However net force

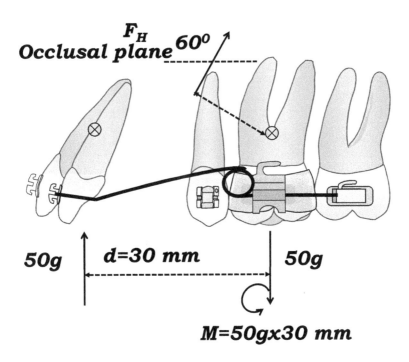

Fig. 12. Biomechanics of incisor intrusion with Burstone's cantilever. Source: Joanna Antoszewska (2009) Wykorzystanie tymczasowego zakotwienia kortykalnego w leczeniu zaburzeń zgryzowo-zębowych. Wrocław : Akad. Med., 5; 111 s. (Rozprawy Habilitacyjne Akademii Medycznej we Wrocławiu). ISBN 978-83-7055-489-7

vector is inclined 60⁰ to the occlusal plane, therefore net force value (F_H) equals: F_H = F_1/sin 60⁰ = 173 g. Furthermore, in order to compensate side effect of Burstone's cantilever - moment inclining molars distally - stripes of high-pull headgear must be attached at the certain distance (D) from the center of molar resistance, thus inclining molars mesially: 50 g x 24h x 30 = 173 g x 8h x D, so D = 26,01 mm. Another example: retraction of front teeth with the 200 g of force simultaneously displaces molars mesially (fig. 13). Horizontal force reinforcing anchorage (F_2) and originating from the low-pull headgear worn 10 hours per day equals 480 g (200 g x 24 h = F_2 x 10 h). Consequently, since the net force vectors of either high-pull as well as low-pull headgears are inclined to the occlusal plane, their efficient force values equal 627 g (480/cos 40⁰) and 679 g (480 g/cos 45⁰) respectively.

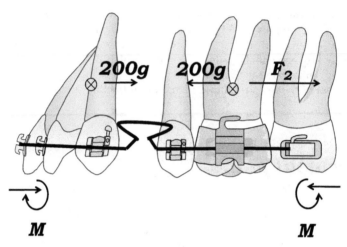

Fig. 13. Biomechanics of controlled space closure. Source: Joanna Antoszewska (2009) Wykorzystanie tymczasowego zakotwienia kortykalnego w leczeniu zaburzeń zgryzowo-zębowych. Wrocław : Akad. Med., 5; 111 s. (Rozprawy Habilitacyjne Akademii Medycznej we Wrocławiu). ISBN 978-83-7055-489-7

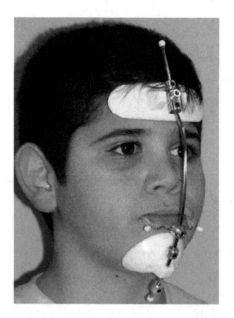

Fig. 14. Face mask

Nevertheless, despite so precise calculations, biologic response is inadequate to the expected one. As reported by Melsen and Bosch[56] when an orthodontic force is applied to a tooth, the cells of periodontal ligaments are differentiated into active osteogenic and osteoclastic cells. As a result, both periodontal ligaments and the adjacent bone exhibit increased cellular activity facilitating tooth movement, therefore headgear - if worn intermittently - is incapable of efficient anchorage reinforcement.

Face mask applied in class III treatment as orthodontic and orthopedic traction (fig. 14) is anchored on a forehead and a chin. Since mandible is a moving structure, therewith its response is unpredictable in terms of mathematic calculations, although efficient clinically. Nevertheless, as anchorage control is also achieved intermittently, all the displacements are resultants of the desired movements and transient collapses.

b. Teeth anchored appliances

Teeth anchored appliances are generally the most popular ones widely used for anchorage reinforcement. Rapid maxillary expander (fig. 15) is an appliance designed to correct transverse discrepancy in class III cases. Nance button - mounted in maxilla and supporting class II correction with eg. repelling magnets[57], superelastic springs[58-60], jones-jig appliance[61-62], pendulum appliance introduced by Hilgers[63] (fig. 16a, b) or Keles slider®[64] (fig. 17) - utilizes hard palate, therefore its efficiency is highly dependent on palatal morphology[65] (fig. 18a, b).

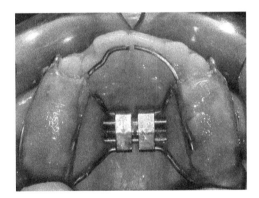

Fig. 15. Rapid maxillary expander

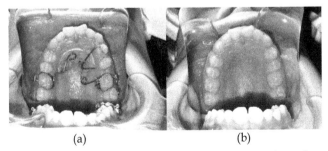

(a)   (b)

Fig. 16. Pendulum appliance: a) inter-dental spaces gained after unilateral activation, b) final symmetric positionof upper molars

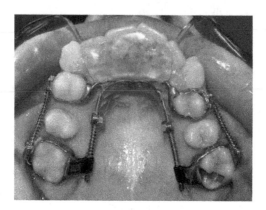

Fig. 17. Keles slider®. Source: Mavropoulos A, Sayinsu K, Allaf F, Kiliaridis S, Papadopoulos MA, Ozlem Keles AO. Noncompliance unilateral maxillary molar distalization. Angle Orthod 2006,3:382-7

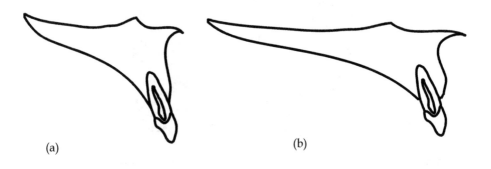

(a)   (b)

Fig. 18. Palatal morphology: a) steep vault and b) flat vaults, respectively favoring and incumbering Nance-button settling. Source: Joanna Antoszewska (2009) Wykorzystanie tymczasowego zakotwienia kortykalnego w leczeniu zaburzeń zgryzowo-zębowych. Wrocław : Akad. Med., 5; 111 s. (Rozprawy Habilitacyjne Akademii Medycznej we Wrocławiu). ISBN 978-83-7055-489-7

On the other hand, bi-maxillary appliances such as Herbst hinge[66] , Carrière distalizer®[67], jasper-jumper[68] (fig. 19a, b), MALU (fig. 20) or Forsus® (Fig. 21a, b), designed for advancement of mandible in young adolescents with concave profile (fig. 22), are dependent on initial teeth-positions. In other terms, protrusion of lower incisors permits functional treatment of class II, since their further flaring is the adverse, unavoidable effect of mandibular forward displacement.

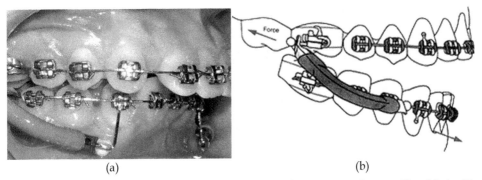

(a)	(b)

Fig. 19. Jasper-jumper a) in situ, b) scheme of delivered force vectors. Source: Küçükkeleş N, Ilhan I, Orgun IA. Treatment efficiency in skeletal Class II patients treated with the jasper jumper. Angle Orthod 2007;77:449-56

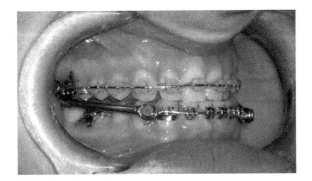

Fig. 20. MALU

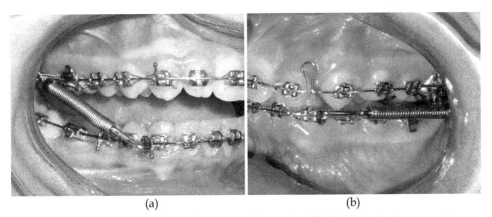

(a)	(b)

Fig. 21. Forsus appliance in situ: a) during mouth opening, b) after mouth closure; note transient class III (over-correction of class II) evident on canines and molars

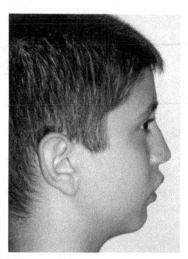

Fig. 22. Concave facial profile of young adolescent – indication for mandibular forward displacement

Evaluating appliances settled on the teeth it may be stated that their biomechanics bases on paradigm that larger overall surface of the roots composing anchor unit is resistant to the orthodontic forces displacing individual tooth (fig. 23). It sounds logic, however this concept is totally opposite to the very interesting one presented by Mulligan and well grounded in terms of biomechanics[69]. The author proved that the undesired molar mesialization during

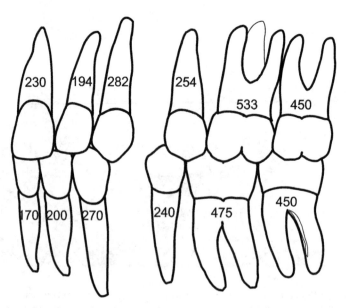

Fig. 23. Periodontal surfaces of each tooth. Source: Proffit W. Contemporary Orthodontics

extraction space closure is independent on periodontal surface of the anchor unit. The only mattering factors are: a) the resilience of the archwire the teeth move along and b) inter-bracket distance from canine to 1st molar. According to this theory, tip-back closest to the mesial margin of a molar-tube rotates anchor tooth-crown distally, whereas magnitude of either force as well as moment acting on canine depend on its distance ("d") from the tip-back bend . If the "d" distance is larger than 2/3 of the inter-bracket distance (fig. 24a), both teeth are subjected to rotating moments of different magnitudes, however of the same direction; thus net rotating moment responsible for anchorage not only has the maximal value, but acts in the direction of canine desired displacement. If the "d" distance equals 2/3 of inter-bracket distance (fig. 24b), although moment rotating favorably exists, however it is not increased with the moment rotating canine distally. Further decrease of the "d" distance" generates rotating moments of the same magnitudes, but of the opposite directions (fig. 24c), uprighting canine root and maintaining molar sagittal position. If such biomechanical standard is embraced, excluding 2nd premolar from the appliance increases the wire resilience and generates higher rotating moments of favorable directions (fig 25a) than including 2nd premolar into the anchor unit (fig. 25b). In other terms, on the contrary to the generally accepted concept, Mulligan's theory proves that decreasing periodontal surface of anchor unit may serve as better anchorage reinforcement.

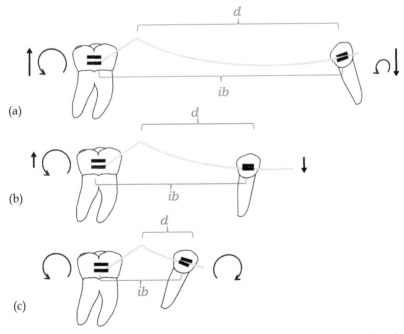

Fig. 24. Forces and moments acting on canine being displaced towards 1st molar, dependent on the distance „d" and inter-bracket distance „ib": a) d>2/3 ib, b) d=2/3 ib, c) d<2/3 ib; note that together with canine distalization (decreasing „d" distance) force value diminishes and moment direction changes after passing a „0" point. Direction of moment acting on canine results from archwire resilience and the distance from 1st molar

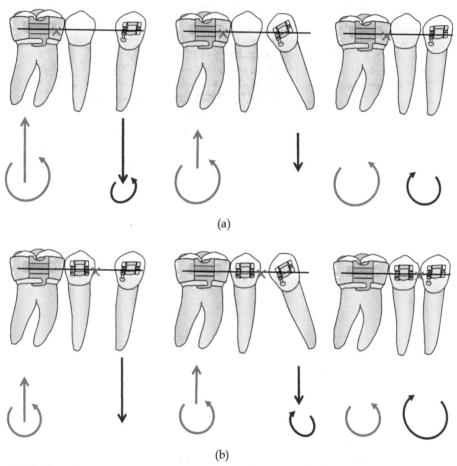

(a)

(b)

Fig. 25. Mulligan's concept: biomechanics of canine distalization if 2nd premolar is: a) excluded from the appliance, b) included in the appliance; "X"-gable bend, moments and forces acting on molars are marked in red, moments and forces acting on canines are marked in blue

2. Current look

Reasons of all the elaborated deliberations are scientifically supported: numerous research upon efficiency and efficacy of conventional anchorage [70-82], directly or indirectly confirm the poorness of their reliability. Despite high prevalence of the appliances reinforcing anchorage - especially in class II treatment - all hitherto discussed devices have certain disadvantages or could not provide anchorage for vertical tooth-movement[83-84]. Furthermore, in the face of overloading periodontal structures possibly leading to root resorption, tissue necrosis or cortical plate atrophy, extra-dental and intraoral source of anchorage has technically become natural point of clinical interest and evaluation: biocompatible implants.

Experimental study began already in 1945, when Gainsforth and Higley[85] introduced vitallium screws to distalize upper teeth (fig. 26). Since they failed (all screws were lost within approximately 1 month), boom for other animal experiments related to implants as anchorage reinforcement falls around turn of 1970 into 1980, after Brånemark and co-workers' success: osseointegration of prosthetic implant and bone. Factors such as alloys used for implant-manufacturing [86,87] as well as resistance to orthodontic loading with forces originating from fixed mechanics[88,89] differentiated the research material. Since the implants succeeded, they were proclaimed as "having the potential to be used as a source of firm osseous anchorage for orthodontics and dentofacial orthopedics"[90].

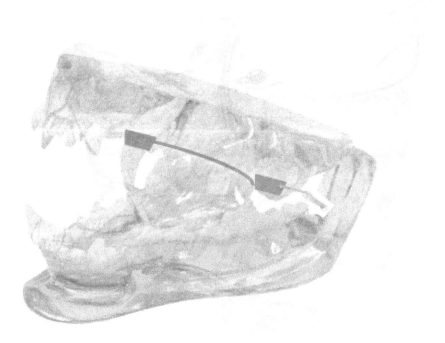

Fig. 26. Study design: Gainsforth and Higley, 1945

Shapiro and Kokich[91] were ones of the pioneers of pre-prosthetic implantation for orthodontic purposes in humans, slowly encouraging other clinicians[92-95]. However, obvious disadvantages of prosthetic implants, such as defeating interadicular placement, complicated surgical procedure associated with insertion, long-lasting osseointegration, biomechanical limitations and high cost were still of a major concern. Such circumstances attracted clinicians' great interest towards "slenderizing" commonly applied screws[96,97] and simplifying their insertion procedures[98] without compromising anchoring properties, thus leading to the development of 21st century orthodontic anchorage: miniscrew implants or TSAD (Temporary Skeletal Anchorage Devices). Their decreased sizes enabled placement in iteradicular spaces of either jaws, for many clinical purposes. Vertical displacements eg. alignment of canted occlusal plane (fig. 27a-c) intrusion of lower incisors (fig. 28a, b) or

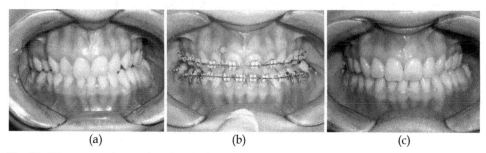

Fig. 27. Alignment of canted occlusal plane using TSAD: a) initial occlusion, b) TSAD loading mode, c) final occlusion

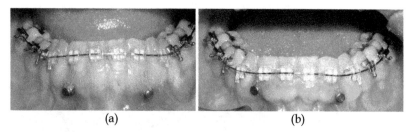

Fig. 28. Intrusion of lower incisors using TSAD: a) prior to TSAD loading, b) final result

lateral teeth (fig. 29a, b), as well as sagittal ones: protraction of lower molars with either sliding (fig. 30a) or segmented mechanics (fig. 30b) have eventually become facilitated and free of side effects. Clinical efficiency encouraged orthodontist to load TSAD multipurposely eg. applying distalizing and intrusive force on continuous (fig. 31a) or segmented (fig. 31b) archwire, extrusive and intrusive forces simultaneously (fig. 32) or even forces acting in three planes of space at the very same moment (fig. 33).

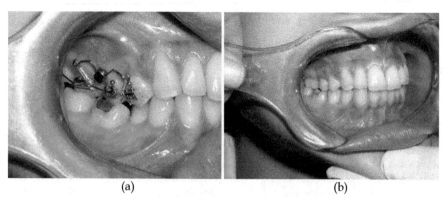

Fig. 29. Intrusion of upper lateral teeth using TSAD: a) prior to TSAD loading, b) final result

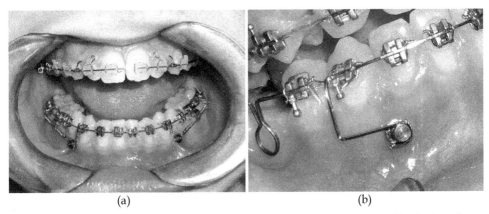

(a)   (b)

Fig. 30. Protraction of lower molars using: a) TSAD and sliding mechanics, b) TSAD and segmented archwires

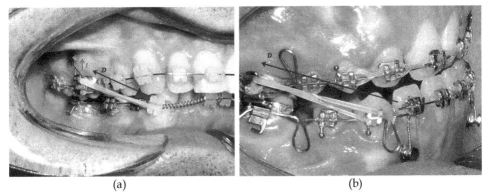

(a)   (b)

Fig. 31. Distalizing (D) and intrusive (I) forces on: a) continuous and b) segmented archwires

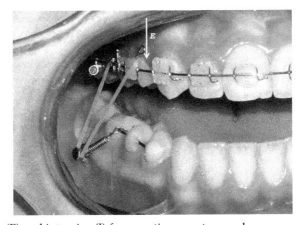

Fig. 32. Extrusive (E) and intrusive (I) forces acting spontaneously

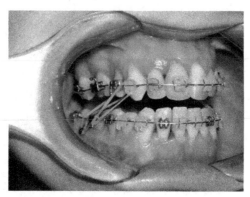

Fig. 33. Transversal, vertical and sagittal forces acting simultaneously

Various practical demands entailed manufacturing and permanent improvement of different miniscrew implant-systems[90,99,100], all the more so that nobody informed about absolute stability (100% success rate) of TSAD. Our routine introducing of the miniscrew implants for anchorage reinforcement in treatment of many types of malocclusion[101-106] allowed us selection of the most versatile and convenient systems: Absoanchor® (Dentos, Daegu, South Corea) and Ortho Easy (Forestadent, Phorzheim, Germany).

Absoanchor® is available as the branch of different diameters, lengths and designs: from 1.2 to 1.6 mm in cross-section, 5 to 12 mm long, cylindrical or tapered, with flat or bracket-like heads, with long, short or no neck. However, in order to make such complex offer less confusing, especially for the beginners we recommend tapered miniscrew implants with small head and convenient hole in the conically-shaped neck; considering lengths and diameters: 6 mm and 1.6 mm in mandible and 8 mm 1.3 mm in maxilla should be chosen for vestibular insertion (fig. 34).

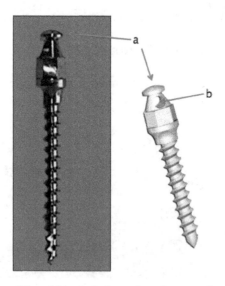

Fig. 34. Absoanchor®: a) small head, b) a hole for utility elements (ligatures, elastomerics)

Ortho Easy pins® are easier to handle: there is only one design available (fig. 35), therefore colour-coded different lengths (pink: 6 mm, violet: 8 mm) simplify the choice dependent on treatment indications and locations in the jaws: short miniscrew implant in mandible, long one in maxilla.

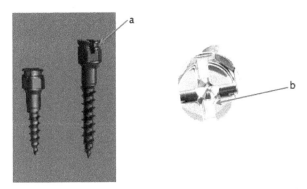

Fig. 35. Ortho Easy pins®: a) undercut facilitating ligating, b) rounded design of slot edges facilitating wire adjustment

Both systems are designed to insert into interadicular space, therefore they may be connected via coil spring with the elements of fixed appliances either bonded to the teeth or attached to the working archwire. It enables loading with forces of mesio-distal direction, so essential in correction of sagittal discrepancies with the vertical component: the most common malocclusions. Direction of the coil spring, dictated by mutual relation of TSAD position and height of attachment (hook) defines the line of force vector (fig. 36a, b).

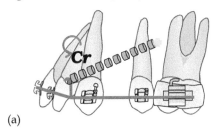

(a)

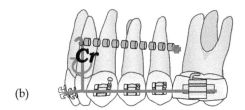

(b)

Fig. 36. Force vectors dependent on mutual relation of TSAD vertical position and height of attachment (hook) on the working archwire: a) rotating moment retruding incisors, b) rotating moment protruding incisors

Forasmuch it is obvious that TSAD position determines biomechanics of orthodontic treatment plan, nobody but orthodontists themselves should insert miniscrew implants. Although there is a myth that bending wires is far beyond the scope of the dentistry, we must not forget we are doctors and if the treatment fails we will be responsible for failures (fig. 37)! The best control is provided by the controller fully aware of the process, thus we would like to encourage our colleagues to become familiar with the details of insertion protocol providing the highest TSAD stability: Wroclaw protocol efficient in 93.43% and obtained after research upon both described TSAD systmes[105-108]. Selection of location for TSAD insertion bases on objective criteria: CT-images at the level of 5 – 7 mm apical of the alveolar crest analyzed by Park et al.[109], visualized the areas of the larger interadicular distances (ID) as well as the ones from the root to the cortical plate (R-CP). According to the provided data, TSAD should be inserted:

1. In maxilla: vestibularly, between central incisors (fig. 38a) or between 2nd bicuspid and 1st molar (fig. 38b) - mean ID = 3.18 mm,
2. In mandible: vestibularly, between 1st and 2nd bicuspids (fig. 39a) - mean ID > 2.20 mm) and between 1st and 2nd molars (fig. 39b) - mean ID = 4.57 mm, mean R-CP = 2.16-5.33 mm; although mean R-CP in mandible progressively increases distally from 1st molar, it is difficult to manipulate in this area, therefore mesial placement seems to be more convenient and still safe.

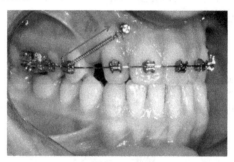

Fig. 37. Improper force vector causing undesired bite opening during planned space closure

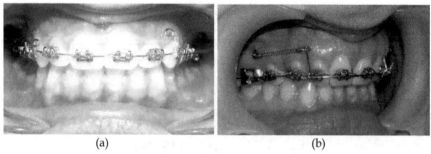

(a)   (b)

Fig. 38. Localization of TSAD in vestibulum of maxilla: a) between central incisors, b) between 2nd premolar and 1st molar; note height of the hook together with vertical position of TSAD form the line of force vector passing above the center of incisor resistance, thus forcing them labially during retraction. Source: Joanna Antoszewska (2009) Wykorzystanie tymczasowego zakotwienia kortykalnego w leczeniu zaburzeń zgryzowo-zębowych. Wrocław : Akad. Med., 5; 111 s. (Rozprawy Habilitacyjne Akademii Medycznej we Wrocławiu). ISBN 978-83-7055-489-7

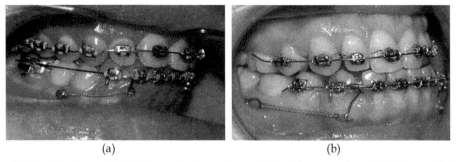

(a)   (b)

Fig. 39. Localization of TSAD in vestibulum of mandible: a) between 1st and 2nd bicuspids, b) between 1st and 2nd molars. Source: Joanna Antoszewska (2009) Wykorzystanie tymczasowego zakotwienia kortykalnego w leczeniu zaburzeń zgryzowo-zębowych. Wrocław : Akad. Med., 5; 111 s. (Rozprawy Habilitacyjne Akademii Medycznej we Wrocławiu). ISBN 978-83-7055-489-7

According to this study, palatal ID between 1st and 2nd molars warrants TSAD stability, however Ludwig et al.[99] in contrast report that anterior part of the palatal bone as the best zone for TSAD insertion (fig. 40). Nevertheless, eg. in case of 2 impacted canines, distal part of palate may serve as suitable area securing TSAD stability (fig. 41). Once the location has been selected, local anesthesia is administered and

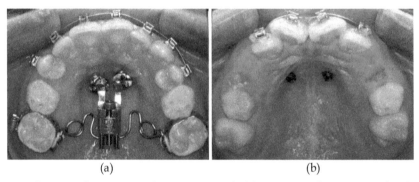

(a)   (b)

Fig. 40. Localization of TSAD on palate recommended by Dr. B. Ludwig; picture by the courtesy of Dr. B. Ludwig

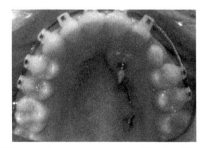

Fig. 41. Localization of TSAD on palate recommended by Prof. Hyo-Sang Park

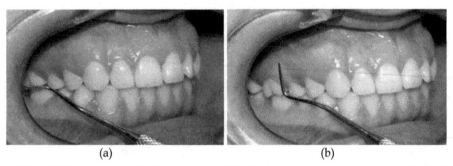

(a)   (b)

Fig. 42. Establishing of interadicular position of TSAD: a) initial position of explorer, b) final position of explorer. Source: Joanna Antoszewska (2009) Wykorzystanie tymczasowego zakotwienia kortykalnego w leczeniu zaburzeń zgryzowo-zębowych. Wrocław : Akad. Med., 5; 111 s. (Rozprawy Habilitacyjne Akademii Medycznej we Wrocławiu). ISBN 978-83-7055-489-7

precise determination of TSAD position takes place. It is accomplished with the dental probe initially oriented parallel to the occlusal plane, with the bend tightly pressed between the crowns of the adjacent teeth with (fig. 42a), then rotated 90^0 towards gingiva (fig. 42b): its tip is located directly in the middle of the interadicular distance. Pressing the tip of explorer firmly against gingiva and oral mucosa causes slight indentation and local ischemia of soft tissues serving as the reference for mesio-distal position of the implant. Vertical position is established along the ischemic line. After vertical, short (4 mm) stab incision, wound margins are pushed aside: this incision is mandatory in order to avoid risk of implementation connective tissue into the screw course during TSAD insertion. Subsequently, a pit is made in cortical plate using a round bur oriented perpendicularly to the bone surface , thus followed with a pilot drill angulated at $30\text{-}40^0$ and $10\text{-}20^0$ to the root axes in maxilla and mandible respectively (fig. 43a, b). This is a pre-drilling method, less forceful for the alveolar process due to significantly lower insertion torque[110], however more time consuming than self-drilling one.

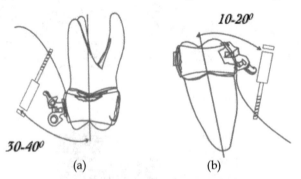

(a)   (b)

Fig. 43. Angulation of Absoanchor®: a) in maxilla, b) in mandible. Source: Joanna Antoszewska (2009) Wykorzystanie tymczasowego zakotwienia kortykalnego w leczeniu zaburzeń zgryzowo-zębowych. Wrocław : Akad. Med., 5; 111 s. (Rozprawy Habilitacyjne Akademii Medycznej we Wrocławiu). ISBN 978-83-7055-489-7

Ambidexterity of an operator, utilized in Wroclaw protocol, secures the most accurate view into the insertion area, with no distortion. Drilling with the speed not exceeding 500 rpm requires massive irrigation to avoid overheating of the bone. The miniscrew implant may be inserted with a manual or engine screw driver, however manual implantation is recommended (especially for the beginners), since during manual insertion orthodontists may notice even minor increase in resistance often related to root contact. If this occurs, it is mandatory to unscrew implant totally and to apply it in a different angulation.

Post-operative inflammation requires no antibiotics[108], however 2-week postponement of loading allows total cease of symptoms.

Periapical radiograms in three projections - perpendicular and two oblique ones to assess root contact recommended by Park[111] are excluded from Wroclaw protocol: one must not neglect neither distortion nor dose protection. In our method, stable position of miniscrew two weeks after insertion indicates no root contact, which allows loading TSAD with initial force value of 50 g, still within primary stability period (fig. 44). This value may be increased accordingly to the treatment needs, after 3 months, up to 180 g per side thus matching data provided by many researchers:

1. forced eruption of impacted tooth: 50g for canine[112] and 80 g for molars[113],
2. intrusion of posterior teeth: 50 g buccolingually per tooth[114], 90 g[115], 100 g[116] or 150-200 g[117],
3. group sagittal movement: 150 g for retraction of 6 front teeth[118] or 180 g[101] for distalization of all upper teeth.

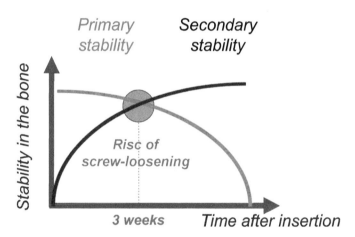

Fig. 44. Diagram illustrating periods of TSAD stability

In serviceable survey of orthodontists[119] evaluation of fear rate before and after TSAD insertion displayed different results. Mean fear level ranked before experiment reached 4.6 and significantly ($p<0.05$) diminished to 3.2 after four trials of TSAD insertion. Factors responsible for fear rate before and after TSAD insertion differed quantitatively and qualitatively (fig. 45). Fear rate before TSAD insertion was mostly associated with risk of injury: dental root (77.14% of clinicians), maxillary sinus (40.00%) or mandibular canal (28.57%). Only few orthodontists submitted other factors such as uncontrolled bur sliding while drilling, breakage of either drill or TSAD, excessive bleeding, soft tissue impaction into the drilled hole, bone necrosis, postoperative complications, and patient's unwilling attitude towards TSAD insertion as well as personal lack of experience. After TSAD insertion, fear rate associated with risk of injury evidently decreased: fear of dental root, maxillary sinus and mandibular canal injuries were submitted by 57.14%, 11.43% and 2.85% of clinicians respectively. Furthermore, spectrum of possibly frightening factors restricted after four trials; besides risk of injury, only uncontrolled bur sliding while drilling remained the fear factor for 2.85% of the surveyed group.

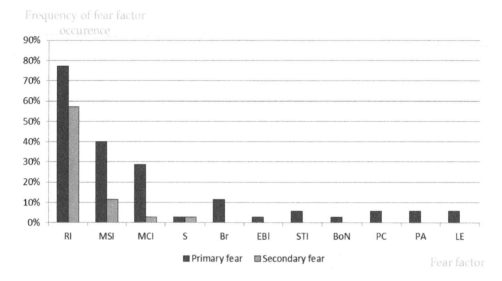

RI - root injury, MSI - maxillary sinus injury, MCI - maxillary canal injury, S - uncontrolled bur sliding while drilling, Br - breakage of either drill or MSI, EBl - excessive bleeding,
STI - soft tissue impaction into the drilled hole, BoN - bone necrosis, PC - postoperative complications,
PA - patient's unwilling attitude towards MSI insertion, LE - lack of experience

Fig. 45. Evaluation of fear rate before and after TSAD insertion. Source: Antoszewska J, Trześniewska P, Kawala B, Ludwig B, Park HS. Qualitative and quantitative evaluation of root injury risk potentially burdening insertion of microscrew implants. Korean J.Orthod. 2011;41,2:112-120

Although TSAD are valuable tools for gaining excellent anchorage, especially in non-compliance patients, their stability is still a problem requiring further investigation. The research of Liou et al.[120] has proven that stable TSAD have not kept their initial position during treatment and tipped even 1.5 mm still serving as an excellent anchorage. Nevertheless establishing risk factors of excessive implant mobility impeding orthodontic force application is crucial for treatment success. So far, the list assessing the highest number of parameters related to TSAD failures, based on the Kaplan–Meier product-limit estimate specifies[105]: low position of the line connecting oral commissures (fig. 46), decreased overbite (fig. 47), Angle class III (fig. 48), vertical location in attached gingiva in mandible (fig. 49), right side of mandible between 1st and 2nd molars (fig. 50), lower molars intrusion and class II traction (fig. 51). Clinical parameters favoring failures are also listed: male sex, age < 20, upper midline shift to the right, centered lower midline and, class III on canines - all of them evident already at the clinical examination, therefore easy to manage and control.

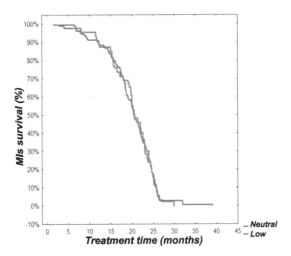

Fig. 46. TSAD stability in relation to position of the line connecting oral commissures: neutral (passing stomion) and low one (beneath stomion). Source: Joanna Antoszewska (2009) Wykorzystanie tymczasowego zakotwienia kortykalnego w leczeniu zaburzeń zgryzowo-zębowych. Wrocław : Akad. Med., 5; 111 s. (Rozprawy Habilitacyjne Akademii Medycznej we Wrocławiu). ISBN 978-83-7055-489-7

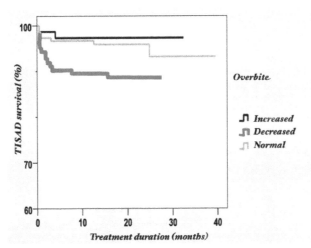

Fig. 47. TSAD stability in relation to an overbite: DB – deep bite, OB – open bite, NOB – normal overbite. Source: Joanna Antoszewska (2009) Wykorzystanie tymczasowego zakotwienia kortykalnego w leczeniu zaburzeń zgryzowo-zębowych. Wrocław : Akad. Med., 5; 111 s. (Rozprawy Habilitacyjne Akademii Medycznej we Wrocławiu). ISBN 978-83-7055-489-7. Source: Antoszewska J, Papadopoulos M, Park HS, Ludwig B. Five-year-experience with orthodontic miniscrew implants: a retrospective investigation of the factors influencing the success rates. Am J Orthod Dentofacial Orthop 2009;136;2:158.e1-158.e10 (on-line), 158-159

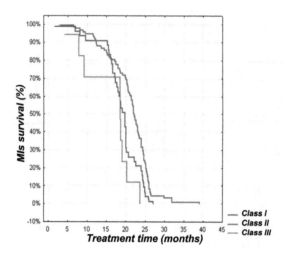

Fig. 48. TSAD stability in relation to the Angle class. Source: Joanna Antoszewska (2009) Wykorzystanie tymczasowego zakotwienia kortykalnego w leczeniu zaburzeń zgryzowo-zębowych. Wrocław : Akad. Med., 5; 111 s. (Rozprawy Habilitacyjne Akademii Medycznej we Wrocławiu). ISBN 978-83-7055-489-7

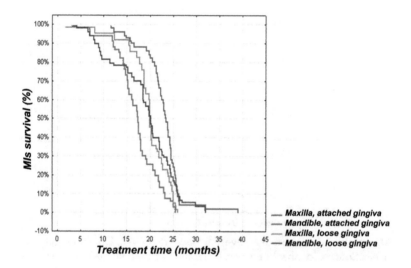

Fig. 49. TSAD stability in relation to its vertical position. Source: Joanna Antoszewska (2009) Wykorzystanie tymczasowego zakotwienia kortykalnego w leczeniu zaburzeń zgryzowo-zębowych. Wrocław : Akad. Med., 5; 111 s. (Rozprawy Habilitacyjne Akademii Medycznej we Wrocławiu). ISBN 978-83-7055-489-7

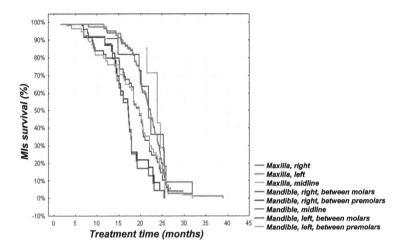

Fig. 50. TSAD stability in relation to its position along the dental arch perimeter. Source: Joanna Antoszewska (2009) Wykorzystanie tymczasowego zakotwienia kortykalnego w leczeniu zaburzeń zgryzowo-zębowych. Wrocław : Akad. Med., 5; 111 s. (Rozprawy Habilitacyjne Akademii Medycznej we Wrocławiu). ISBN 978-83-7055-489-7

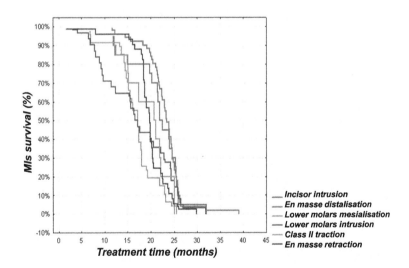

Fig. 51. TSAD stability in relation to orthodontic displacement. Source: Joanna Antoszewska (2009) Wykorzystanie tymczasowego zakotwienia kortykalnego w leczeniu zaburzeń zgryzowo-zębowych. Wrocław : Akad. Med., 5; 111 s. (Rozprawy Habilitacyjne Akademii Medycznej we Wrocławiu). ISBN 978-83-7055-489-7

Considering rate of stability, certainly mini plates prevail over single miniscrew implants, however the former ones demand on more complex surgical protocol[121-126]. Nevertheless, rapid development of orthodontic anchorage design as well as progressively increasing interest of practitioners towards application of mini plates in mostly simple manner already provoked the positive feedback: system addressed to orthodontists only[127-134].

Summing up, miniscrew implants and mini plates increasing popularity among clinicians is quite likely to displace conventional appliances for anchorage reinforcement, therefore "gravity center" of knowledge provided in this chapter has been moved towards details of planning and application of temporary skeletal anchorage devices.

3. References

[1] Tweed Ch. Indications for the extraction of teeth in orthodontic procedure. Am J Orthod Oral Surg. 1944-1945;42:22-45.

[2] Levrini A, Favero L. The masters of functional orthodontics. 2003, Quintessence Publishing, New Malden, Surrey, UK.

[3] McLaughlin RP, Bennett JC, Trevisi H. Systematized orthodontic treatment mechanics. 2001, second edition, Mosby International Ltd.

[4] Gandini LG Jr, Gandini MR, Amaral RM. Continuous torque system with control of the reaction unit. Am J Orthod Dentofacial Orthop. 2010;137:393-5.

[5] Viecilli RF. Self-corrective T-loop design for differential space closure. Am J Orthod Dentofacial Orthop. 2006;129:48-53.

[6] Choy K, Pae EK, Kim KH, Park YC, Burstone CJ. Controlled space closure with a statically determinate retraction system. Angle Orthod. 2002;72:191-8.

[7] Kuhlberg AJ, Burstone CJ. T-loop position and anchorage control. Am J Orthod Dentofacial Orthop. 1997;112:12-8.

[8] Shroff B, Yoon WM, Lindauer SJ, Burstone CJ. Simultaneous intrusion and retraction using a three-piece base arch. Angle Orthod.1997;67:455-61.

[9] Kalra V, Burstone CJ, Nanda R. More on fixed magnetic appliances. Am J Orthod Dentofacial Orthop. 1990;97:27A-28A.

[10] Manhartsberger C, Morton JY, Burstone CJ. Space closure in adult patients using the segmented arch technique. Angle Orthod. 1989;59:205-10.

[11] Burstone CJ. The segmented arch approach to space closure. Am J Orthod. 1982;82:361-78.

[12] Park JH, Cruz C, Alexander RG. An orthodontic/orthopedic correction of the Class III malocclusion in young patients with a modified RPE appliance and a facemask. Int J Orthod Milwaukee. 2010;21:23-6.

[13] Isci D, Turk T, Elekdag-Turk S. Activation-deactivation rapid palatal expansion and reverse headgear in Class III cases. Eur J Orthod. 2010;32:706-15. Epub 2010 May 9.

[14] León-Salazar V, Janson G, de Freitas MR, de Almeida RR, León-Salazar R. Nonextraction treatment of a skeletal Class III malocclusion. Am J Orthod Dentofacial Orthop. 2009;136:736-45.

[15] Hamamci N, Başaran G, Tümen EC, Ozdemir E. Nonsurgical orthodontic treatment of an adolescent girl with Class III malocclusion and asymmetric maxillary narrowing. Am J Orthod Dentofacial Orthop. 2008;134:309-17.

[16] Baccetti T, Rey D, Angel D, Oberti G, McNamara JA Jr. Mandibular cervical headgear vs rapid maxillary expander and facemask for orthopedic treatment of Class III malocclusion. Angle Orthod. 2007;77:619-24.

[17] Pangrazio-Kulbersh V, Berger JL, Janisse FN, Bayirli B. Long-term stability of Class III treatment: rapid palatal expansion and protraction facemask vs LeFort I maxillary advancement osteotomy. Am J Orthod Dentofacial Orthop. 2007;131:7.e9-19.

[18] Kama JD, Ozer T, Baran S. Orthodontic and orthopaedic changes associated with treatment in subjects with Class III malocclusions. Eur J Orthod. 2006;28:496-502. Epub 2006 Jun 13.

[19] Arman A, Ufuk Toygar T, Abuhijleh E. Evaluation of maxillary protraction and fixed appliance therapy in Class III patients. Eur J Orthod. 2006;28:383-92. Epub 2006 May 26.

[20] Liou EJ. Effective maxillary orthopedic protraction for growing Class III patients: a clinical application simulates distraction osteogenesis. Prog Orthod. 2005;6:154-71.

[21] Arslan SG, Kama JD, Baran S. Correction of a severe Class III malocclusion. Am J Orthod Dentofacial Orthop. 2004;126:237-44.

[22] Westwood PV, McNamara JA Jr, Baccetti T, Franchi L, Sarver DM. Long-term effects of Class III treatment with rapid maxillary expansion and facemask therapy followed by fixed appliances. Am J Orthod Dentofacial Orthop. 2003;123:306-20.

[23] Cha KS. Skeletal changes of maxillary protraction in patients exhibiting skeletal class III malocclusion: a comparison of three skeletal maturation groups. Angle Orthod. 2003;73:26-35.

[24] Keles A, Tokmak EC, Erverdi N, Nanda R. Effect of varying the force direction on maxillary orthopedic protraction. Angle Orthod. 2002;72:387-96.

[25] Baccetti T, Franchi L, McNamara JA Jr. Treatment and posttreatment craniofacial changes after rapid maxillary expansion and facemask therapy. Am J Orthod Dentofacial Orthop. 2000;118:404-13.

[26] Lima Filho RM, de Oliveira Ruellas AC. Long-term maxillary changes in patients with skeletal Class II malocclusion treated with slow and rapid palatal expansion. Am J Orthod Dentofacial Orthop. 2008;134:383-8.

[27] Lima Filho RM, Ruellas AC. Long-term anteroposterior and vertical maxillary changes in skeletal class II patients treated with slow and rapid maxillary expansion. Angle Orthod. 2007;77:870-4.

[28] Lima Filho RM, de Oliveira Ruellas AC. Mandibular behavior with slow and rapid maxillary expansion in skeletal Class II patients: a long-term study. Angle Orthod. 2007;77:625-31.

[29] Frye L, Diedrich PR, Kinzinger GS. Class II treatment with fixed functional orthodontic appliances before and after the pubertal growth peak – a cephalometric study to evaluate differential therapeutic effects. J Orofac Orthop. 2009;70:511-27.

[30] Siara-Olds NJ, Pangrazio-Kulbersh V, Berger J, Bayirli B. Long-term dentoskeletal changes with the Bionator, Herbst, Twin Block, and MARA functional appliances. Angle Orthod. 2010;80:18-29.

[31] Chaiyongsirisern A, Rabie AB, Wong RW. Stepwise advancement Herbst appliance versus mandibular sagittal split osteotomy. Treatment effects and long-term stability of adult Class II patients. Angle Orthod. 2009;79:1084-94.

[32] Panigrahi P, Vineeth V. Biomechanical effects of fixed functional appliance on craniofacial structures. Angle Orthod. 2009;79:668-75.

[33] Kinzinger G, Frye L, Diedrich P. Class II treatment in adults: comparing camouflage orthodontics, dentofacial orthopedics and orthognathic surgery – a cephalometric study to evaluate various therapeutic effects. J Orofac Orthop. 2009;70:63-91. Epub 2009 Feb 5.

[34] Sloss EA, Southard KA, Qian F, Stock SE, Mann KR, Meyer DL, Southard TE. Comparison of soft-tissue profiles after treatment with headgear or Herbst appliance. Am J Orthod Dentofacial Orthop. 2008;133:509-14.

[35] Giannasi LC, Magini M, de Oliveira CS, de Oliveira LV. Treatment of obstructive sleep apnea using an adjustable mandibular repositioning appliance fitted to a total prosthesis in a maxillary edentulous patient. Sleep Breath. 2008;12:91-5.

[36] Naini FB, Gill DS, Payne E, Keel B. Medium Opening Activator: design, applications for the management of class II deep overbite malocclusion. World J Orthod. 2007;8:e1-9.

[37] VanLaecken R, Martin CA, Dischinger T, Razmus T, Ngan P. Treatment effects of the edgewise Herbst appliance: a cephalometric and tomographic investigation. Am J Orthod Dentofacial Orthop. 2006;130:582-93.

[38] Kinzinger G, Gülden N, Roth A, Diedrich P. Disc-condyle relationships during class II Treatment with the functional mandibular advancer (FMA). J Orofac Orthop. 2006;67:356-75.

[39] Bass NM. The Dynamax system: a new orthopaedic appliance and case report. J Orthod. 2006;33:78-89.

[40] Shen G, Hägg U, Darendeliler M. Skeletal effects of bite jumping therapy on the mandible - removable vs. fixed functional appliances. Orthod Craniofac Res.2005;8:2-10.

[41] Voudouris JC, Woodside DG, Altuna G, Angelopoulos G, Bourque PJ, Lacouture CY, Kuftinec MM. Condyle-fossa modifications and muscle interactions during Herbst treatment, Part 2. Results and conclusions. Am J Orthod Dentofacial Orthop. 2003;124:13-29.

[42] Voudouris JC, Woodside DG, Altuna G, Kuftinec MM, Angelopoulos G, Bourque PJ. Condyle-fossa modifications and muscle interactions during herbst treatment, part 1: new technological methods. Am J Orthod Dentofacial Orthop. 2003;123:604-13.

[43] Kinzinger G, Ostheimer J, Förster F, Kwandt PB, Reul H, Diedrich P. Development of a new fixed functional appliance for treatment of skeletal class II malocclusion first report. J Orofac Orthop. 2002;63:384-99.

[44] Dolce C, Van Sickels JE, Bays RA, Rugh JD. Skeletal stability after mandibular advancement with rigid versus wire fixation. J Oral Maxillofac Surg. 2000;58:1219-27.

[45] Blomqvist JE, Isaksson S. Skeletal stability after mandibular advancement: a comparison of two rigid internal fixation techniques. J Oral Maxillofac Surg. 1994;52:1133-7.

[46] Sadowsky C, Schneider BJ, BeGole EA, Tahir E. Long-term stability after orthodontic treatment: nonextraction with prolonged retention. Am J Orthod Dentofacial Orthop. 1994;106:243-9.

[47] Newton I. Philosophiae Naturalis Principia Mathematica, 1687, S. Pepys, Reg. Sor. Praeses, London.

[48] Melsen B, Fotis V, Burstone CJ. Vertical force considerations in differential space closure. J Clin Orthod. 1990;24:678-83.

[49] Sifakakis I, Pandis N, Makou M, Eliades T, Bourauel C. Forces and moments on posterior teeth generated by incisor intrusion biomechanics. Orthod Craniofac Res. 2009;12:305-11.

[50] Badawi HM, Toogood RW, Carey JP, Heo G, Major PW. Three-dimensional orthodontic force measurements. Am J Orthod Dentofacial Orthop. 2009;136:518-28.

[51] Cattaneo PM, Dalstra M, Melsen B. Moment-to-force ratio, center of rotation, and force level: a finite element study predicting their interdependency for simulated orthodontic loading regimens. Am J Orthod Dentofacial Orthop. 2008;133:681-9.

[52] Proffit WR, Fields HW Jr., Sarver DM. Contemporary Orthodontics. 2006, Elsevier Health Sciences, Edition 4.

[53] Teuscher UM. An appraisal of growth and reaction to extraoral anchorage. Am J Orthod 1986;89:113-21.

[54] Schmuth GPF, Holtgrave EA, Drescher DISBN: 83-87601-20-9, Czelej, Wydanie 1,

[55] Braun S. Extraoral appliances: a twenty-first century update. Am J Orthod Dentofacial Orthop 2004;125:624-9.

[56] Melsen B, Bosch C. Different approaches to anchorage: a survey and evaluation. Angle Orthod 1997;67;1:23-30.

[57] Steger ES, Blechman AM. Case reports: molar distalization with static repelling magnets. Part II. Am J Orthod Dentofacial Orthop 1995;108:547-55.

[58] Bondemark L. A comparative analysis of distal maxillary molar movement produced by a new lingual intra-arch coil appliance and magnetic appliance. Eur J Orthod 2000;22:683-95.

[59] Dunin-Wilczyńska I. Jednostronna dystalizacja pierwszego trzonowca górnego sprężyną ściśniętą. Ortod. Współcz. 2001;3;2:37-9.

[60] Gulati S, Kharbanda OP, Parkash H. Dental and skeletal changes after intra-oral molar distalization with sectional jig assembly. Am J Orthod Dentofacial Orthop 1998;114:319-27.

[61] Bolla E, Muratore F, Carano A, Bowman SJ. Evaluation of Maxillary Molar Distalization With the Distal Jet: A Comparison With Other Contemporary Methods. The Angle Orthodontist: October 2002, Vol. 72, No. 5, pp. 481-94.

[62] Paul LD, O'Brien KD, Mandall NA. Upper removable appliance or jones jig for distalizing first molars? A randomized clinical trial. Orthod Craniofacial Res 2002;5:238-42.

[63] Hilgers JJ. The pendulum appliance for class II non-compliance therapy. J Clin Orthod 1992;67:249-71.

[64] Keles A. Maxillary unilateral distalization with sliding mechanics. Eur J Orthod 2001;23:507-15.

[65] Roberts-Harry D, Sandy J. Orthodontics. Part 9: anchorage control and distal movement. British Dent J 2004;196;5:255-63.

[66] Pancherz H, Anehus-Pancherz M. The head-gear effect of the Herbst appliance. A cephalometric long-term study. Am J Orthod Dentofacial Orthop 1993;103:510-20.

[67] Carrière L. A new Class II distalizer. J Clin Orthod 2004;38:224-31.

[68] Küçükkeleş N, Ilhan I, Orgun IA. Treatment efficiency in skeletal Class II patients treated with the jasper jumper. Angle Orthod 2007;77:449-56.

[69] Mulligan TF. Common sense mechanics in everyday orthodontics. 2009, CSM Publishing, Phoenix, Arizona, USA.

[70] Lloyd TG, Stephens CD. Spontaneous changes in molar occlusion after extraction of all first premolars: a study of class II/1 cases treated with removable appliances. Br J Orth 1979;6:91-4.

[71] Stephens CD, Lloyd TG. Changes in molar occlusion after extraction of all first premolars: a follow up study of class II/1 cases treated with removable appliances. Br J Orth 1980;7:139-44.

[72] Taner TU, Yukay F., Pehlivanoglu M, Çakirer B. A comparative analysis of maxillary tooth movement produced by cervical headgear and pend-x appliance. Angle Orthod 2003;73:686-91.

[73] Rudge SJ. A simplified method of applying extra-oral anchorage. Br Dent J 1981;152:205-6.

[74] Ghosh J, Nanda RS. Evaluation of intramolar distalization technique. Am J Orthod Dentofacial Orthop 1996;110:639-46.

[75] Byloff FK, Darandeliler MA. Distal molar movement using the pendulum appliance. Angle Orthod 1997;67:249-60.

[76] Bondemark L, Kurol J. Class II correction with magnets and super-elastic coils followed by straight-wire mechanotherapy. J Orofacial Orthop 1998;59:127-38.

[77] Alwali S, Marklund M, Persson M. Apical root resorption of upper first molars as related to anchorage system. Swed Dent J 2000;24:145-53.

[78] Bolla E, Muratore F, Carano A, Bowman J. Evaluation of maxillary molar distalization with the distal jet: a comparison with other temporary methods. Angle Orthod 2002;72:481-94.

[79] Brickman CD, Siha PK, Nanda RS. Evaluation of the jones jig appliance for distal molar movement. Am J Orthod Dentofacial Orthop 2000;118:526-34.

[80] Chiu PP. A comparison of two intraoral molar distalization appliances: distal jet versus pendulum appliance [unpublished master's thesis]. Ann Arbor, Mich: Department of Orthodontics, University of Michigan, 2001.

[81] Langlade M. Clinical distalization with the distalix. World J Orthod 2003;4:215-28.

[82] Paul LD, O'Brien KD, Mandall NA. Upper removable appliance or jones jig for distalizing first molars? A randomized clinical trial. Orthod Craniofacial Res 2002;5:238-42.

[83] Firouz M, Zernik J, Nanda R.: Dental and orthopedic effects of high-pull headgear in treatment of class II division 1 malocclusion. Am J Orthod Dentofacial Orthop 1992;102:197-205.

[84] Ng J, Major P, Flores-Mir C. True molar intrusion attained during orthodontic treatment. Am J Orthod Dentofacial Orthop 2006;130:709-14.

[85] Gainsforth BL, Higley LB. A study of orthodontic anchorage possibilities in basal bone. Am J Orthod Oral Surg 1945;31:406-17.

[86] Sherman AJ. Bone reaction to orthodontic forces or vitreous carbon dental implants. Am J Orthod 1978;74:79-87.

[87] Smith JR. Bone dynamics associated with the controlled loading of bioglass-coated aluminum endosteal implants. Am J Orthod 1979;76:618-36.

[88] Majzoub Z, Finotti M, Miotti F, Giardino R, Cordioli G. Bone response to orthodontic loading of endosseous implants in the rabbit calvaria. Early continuous distalizing forces. Eur J Orthod 1999;21:223-30

[89] Roberts WE, Smith RK, Zilberman Y, Mozsary PG, Smith RS. Osseous adaptation to continuous loading of rigid endosseous implants. Am J Orthod 1984;86:95-111.

[90] Sung J.H., Kyung H.M., Bae S.M., Park H.S., Kwon O.W., McNamara J.A.: Microimplants in orthodontics. Daegu: Dentos 2006.

[91] Shapiro PA, Kokich VG. Use of implants in orthodontics. Dent Clin North Am 1988;32:539-50.

[92] Roberts WE, Nelson CL, Goodacre CJ. Rigid implant anchorage to close a mandibular first molar extraction site. J Clin Orthod 1994;28:693-704.

[93] Block MS, Hoffman DR. A new device of absolute anchorage for orthodontics. Am J Orthod Dentofacial Orthop 1995;107:251-8.

[94] Hong H, Ngan P, Li HG, Qi LG, Wei SHY. Use of onplants as stable anchorage for facemask treatment: a case report. Angle Orthod2005;75:453-60.

[95] Janssesns F, Swennen G, Dujardin T, Glineur R, Malevez C. Use of onplants as orthodontic anchorage. Am J Orthod Dentofacial Orthop 2002;122:566-70.

[96] Creekmore TD, Eklund MK. The possibility of skeletal anchorage. J Clin Orthod 1983;17:266-9.

[97] Kanomi R. Mini-implant for orthodontic anchorage. Int J Clin Orthod 1997;31:763-7.

[98] Costa A, Raffini M, Melsen B. Microscrew as orthodontic anchorage. Int J Adult Orthod Orthognath Surg 1998;13:201-9.

[99] Ludwig B., Baumgaertel S., Bowman S.J.: Mini-implants in orthodontics.   Berlin: Quintesence 2008.

[100] Cheol-Ho Paik CH, Park IK, Woo Y, Kim TW. Orthodontic miniscrew implants, clinical applications. 2008 Mosby.

[101] Antoszewska J. Class II division 2 treatment supported by absolute anchorage - case report. Dent. Med. Probl. 2007;44;2:275-80.

[102] Antoszewska J. Mikroimplanty systemu Absoanchor w leczeniu zgryzu otwartego - opis przypadku. Ortod. Pol. 2007;1;1:23-8.

[103] Antoszewska J, Minch L. Literature-based clinical application of microimplants in treatment of different malocclusions. Dent. Med. Probl. 2006 43;1:11-4.

[104] Antoszewska J, Sarul M, Kawala B. Asymetryczna dystalizacja zębów szczęki w oparciu o mikroimplanty Absoanchor.   Opis przypadku. Implantoprotetyka 2008;9;4:25-8.

[105] Antoszewska J. Wykorzystanie tymczasowego zakotwienia kortykalnego w leczeniu zaburzeń zgryzowo-zębowych. 2009, Wrocław Medical University, habilitation thesis ISBN 978-83-7055-489-7.

[106] Antoszewska J, Papadopoulos M, Park HS, Ludwig B. Five-year-experience with orthodontic miniscrew implants: a retrospective investigation of the factors influencing the success rates. Am J Orthod Dentofacial Orthop 2009;136;2:158.e1-158.e10 (on- line), 158-159.

[107] Antoszewska J, Kawala B, Sarul M. Factors affecting stability of orthodontic implants. A Wroclaw method Forum Ortodont. 2010;6,1:5-14.

[108] Antoszewska J, Szeląg J. Pharmacotherapy in orthodontic treatment supported by micro-implants. Pharmacol Rep 2007;59;1:254-6.

[109] Park HS. An anatomical study using CT images for the implantation of micro-implants. Korea J Ortho 2002;32:435-41.

[110] Florvaag B, Kneuertz P, Lazar F, Koebke J, Zöller JE, Braumann B, Mischkowski RA.J Orofac Orthop. Biomechanical properties of orthodontic miniscrews. An in-vitro study. J Orofac Orthop. 2010;71:53-67. Epub 2010 Feb 5.

[111] Park HS. The skeletal cortical anchorage using titanium microscrew implants. Korea J. Orthod. 1999, 29:699-706.

[112] Park HS, Oh YH. Forced eruption of a labially impacted canine using joined micro-implants. J Clin Orthod. 2010;44:108-13; quiz 106.

[113] Janssens F, Swennen G, Dujardin T, Glineur R, Malevez C. Use of an onplant as orthodontic anchorage. Am J Orthod Dentofacial Orthop 2002;122:566-70.

[114] Melsen B, Fiorelli G. Upper molar intrusion. J Clin Orthod 1996;30:91-6.

[115] Kalra V, Burstone CJ, Nanda R. Effects of a fixed magnetic appliance on the dentofacial complex. Am J Orthod Dentofacial Orthop 1989;95:467-78.

[116] Moon CH, Wee JU, Lee HS. Intrusion of overerupted molars by corticotomy and orthodontic skeletal anchorage. Angle Orthod. 2007;77:1119-25.

[117] Park YC, Lee SY, Kim DH, Jee SH. Intrusion of posterior teeth using mini-screw implants. Am J Orthod Dentofacial Orthop 2003;123:690-4.

[118] Park HS, Kwon TG. Sliding mechanics with microscrew implant anchorage. Angle Orthod. 2004;74:703-10.

[119] Antoszewska J, Trześniewska P, Kawala B, Park HS. Qualitative and quantitative evaluation of root injury risk potentially burdening insertion of microscrew implants. Korean J.Orthod. 2011;41,2:112-120.

[120] Liou EJ, Pai BC, Lin JC. Do miniscrews remain stationary under orthodontic forces? Am J Orthod Dentofacial Orthop 2004;126:42-7.

[121] Choi BH, Zhu SJ, Kim YH. A clinical evaluation of titanium miniplates as anchors for orthodontic treatment. Am J Orthod Dentofacial Orthop 2005;128:382-4.

[122] Kärcher H, Byloff FK, Clar E. The Graz implant supported pendulum. A technical note. J Craniomaxillofac Surg 2002;30:87-90.

[123] Sugawara J, Daimaruya T, Umemori M, Nagasaka H, Takahashi I, Kawamura H., Mitani H.: Distal movement of mandibular molars in adult patients with the skeletal anchorage system. Am J Orthod Dentofacial Orthop. 2004;125:130-8.

[124] De Clerck HJ, Cornelis MA, Cevidanes LH, Heymann GC, Tulloch CJF. Orthopedic Traction of the Maxilla With Miniplates: A New Perspective for Treatment of Midface Deficiency. J Oral Maxillofac Surg 2009, 67: 2123-9.

[125] Sugawara J, Aymach Z, Nagasaka DH, Kawamura H, Nanda R. "Surgery first" orthognathics to correct a skeletal class II malocclusion with an impinging bite. J Clin Orthod. 2010;44:429-38.

[126] Nagasaka H, Sugawara J, Kawamura H, Nanda R. "Surgery first" skeletal Class III correction using the Skeletal Anchorage System. J Clin Orthod. 2009;43:97-105.

[127] Kim SH, Kang SM, Choi YS, Kook YA, Chung KR, Huang JC. Cone-beam computed tomography evaluation of mini-implants after placement: Is root proximity a major risk factor for failure? Am J Orthod Dentofacial Orthop. 2010;138:264-76.

[128] Chung KR, Kim SH, Choo H, Kook YA, Cope JB. Distalization of the mandibular dentition with mini-implants to correct a Class III malocclusion with a midline deviation. Am J Orthod Dentofacial Orthop. 2010;137:135-46.

[129] Kim SH, Kook YA, Jeong DM, Lee W, Chung KR, Nelson G. Clinical application of accelerated osteogenic orthodontics and partially osseointegrated mini-implants for minor tooth movement. Am J Orthod Dentofacial Orthop. 2009;136:431-9.

[130] Kim SH, Kook YA, Lee W, Kim I, Chung KR. Two-component mini-implant as an efficient tool for orthognathic patients. Am J Orthod Dentofacial Orthop. 2009;135:110-7.

[131] Chung KR, Kim SH, Kook YA, Kang YG, Sinclair PM. Dental midline correction using two component C-orthodontic mini-implant. Prog Orthod. 2009;10:76-86.

[132] Kim SH, Cho JH, Chung KR, Kook YA, Nelson G. Removal torque values of surface-treated mini-implants after loading. Am J Orthod Dentofacial Orthop. 2008;134:36-43.

[133] Chung KR, Kim SH, Kook YA, Son JH. Anterior torque control using partial-osseointegrated mini-implants: biocreative therapy type I technique. World J Orthod. 2008;9:95-104.

[134] Chung K, Kim SH, Kook Y. C-orthodontic microimplant for distalization of mandibular dentition in Class III correction. Angle Orthod. 2005;75:119-28.

7

Neural Modulation of Orthodontic Tooth Movement

John K. Neubert, Robert M. Caudle, Calogero Dolce, Edgardo J. Toro,
Yvonne Bokrand-Donatelli and L. Shannon Holliday
University of Florida College of Dentistry
United States of America

1. Introduction

Millions of people worldwide have orthodontic therapy for the treatment of dental malocclusions, craniofacial disorders, and simply to improve their appearance. However, orthodontic treatment has several major problems, including the long time braces must be worn, the pain involved during treatment, and the need to wear retainers to prevent relapse. Orthodontics could be improved. Understanding the mechanisms involved with orthodontic tooth movement represents a first step toward this goal. Improvements in the practice of orthodontics would have an immediate and significant impact on the millions of individuals undergoing orthodontic treatment worldwide.

Orthodontic tooth movement can be thought of as an interaction of mechanical force on biological tissue (Krishnan and Davidovitch, 2006; Wise and King, 2008). Much progress in orthodontics has involved finding better means to apply mechanical force to teeth. While advances have been made regarding the mechanics and materials used in orthodontics, there has been a relative plateau in the overall treatment outcomes. For example, a moderately difficult case still requires an average of 18-36 months for treatment, no different than 50 years ago. It is apparent that discoveries relating to biological manipulations may provide a path for significantly improving orthodontic practice.

It is thought that enhancing the speed of orthodontic tooth movement could be accomplished if bone remodeling occurred at an accelerated rate in the alveolar bone associated with the teeth being moved. While this has not been formally demonstrated in the clinic, animal studies strongly support this notion. For example, orthodontic tooth movement in a mouse model was accelerated by overexpressing Receptor Activator of Nuclear Factor Kappa B-Ligand (RANKL) (Kanzaki et al., 2006). RANKL promotes the formation and bone resorptive activity of osteoclasts, the specialized cells charged with bone resorption (Hofbauer and Heufelder, 2001). Conversely, inhibitors of osteoclast formation and activity including osteoprotegerin (OPG), integrin inhibitors, bisphosphonates and inhibitors of matrix metalloproteinases all slowed tooth movement (Holliday et al., 2003; Dolce et al., 2003; Kanzaki et al., 2004; Dunn et al., 2007). Although these studies showed that it is possible to manipulate the speed at which orthodontic tooth movement proceeds by altering osteoclast activity, the specific agents tested to date are probably inappropriate for orthodontic use in the clinic as there would be too much danger of off target effects. Such risks are unacceptable for orthodontic procedures. Although orthodontics as currently practiced is imperfect, it is quite effective. Moreover, children are the most common patients in the orthodontic clinic; for biological manipulations to enhance orthodontics to be contemplated, they must be very safe.

Biological manipulation might be useful in orthodontics to prevent relapse. It is possible that enhancers of bone formation rates might be used to remodel alveolar bone to reduce incidence of relapse and minimize the use of retainers. In this case, it is possible that uncoupled stimulators of bone formation (ie regulation that stimulates bone formation without corresponding bone resorption) might prove ideal. As will be described below, modulators of sclerostin signaling, or other regulators of the Wnt-signaling pathway, are obvious candidates for this application (Paszty et al., 2010; Moester et al., 2010).

Pain is accepted as a necessary off target effect of orthodontics, and is typically treated using common non-prescription pain medications like acetaminophen. For theoretical reasons acetaminophen, which acts centrally, is considered better than ibuprophen or aspirin, which act on prostaglandins locally (Simmons and Brandt, 1992; Kehoe et al., 1996; Walker and Buring, 2001). After an initial period of discomfort (a few days) pain goes away until the next activation of the appliance. The initial activation is usually considered the most painful. In general, orthodontic pain has been considered manageable and acceptable to patients, or at least to the patient's parents, as a necessary component of orthodontic treatment. For this reason, despite its widespread use, relatively little effort has been expended to identify ways to reduce orthodontic pain. Interestingly, as more adults are undergoing orthodontic treatment, more attention has been paid to means for relieving orthodontic pain.

It is thought that pain can be reduced by modifying orthodontic procedures, particularly by using lighter forces to cause less damage and inflammation. Treatment of orthodontic pain is complicated by the fact that tooth movement may require inflammation, triggered by mechanical damage to tissues of the periodontal ligament (PDL) and associated alveolar bone, which is caused by the application of orthodontic force. Efforts to reduce the inflammation either by reducing force or by using local anti-inflammatory agents may compromise the process of tooth movement (Simmons and Brandt, 1992; Kehoe et al., 1996; Walker and Buring, 2001). In fact, there are very few studies that objectively address any of these questions in humans or even in animal models (Bergius et al., 2000; Giannopoulou et al., 2006; Eversole, 2006). For example, there currently are no animal models for studying levels of orthodontic force compared with levels of pain and the amount of tooth movement. Without proper studies, opinions on pain in orthodontics are now based largely on anecdotal evidence.

Orthodontic tooth movement is more complicated than simply applying force, causing mechanical damage and inflammation, followed by bone resorption as part of the response to inflammation and damage. Orthodontic tooth movement requires the presence of a functional PDL (Krishnan and Davidovitch, 2006; Wise and King, 2008). Ankylosed teeth do not move regardless of the amount of force applied to the tooth, or the amount of inflammation induced. The precise mechanisms by which the PDL transduces force to stimulate bone resorption to allow for movement of a tooth through bone are still mysterious. For example, it is known that RANKL is expressed at higher levels on the pressure side of a tooth, but the mechanism supporting the increased RANKL expression is not known.

Recent data demonstrate previously unsuspected links between the neural system and bone remodeling and offer potential strategies for improving orthodontic treatment. Taking advantage of these opportunities requires understanding in greater detail how the neural system is involved in the regulation of orthodontic tooth movement. Neurons and the bone cells involved in the remodelling required for orthodontic tooth movement share numerous molecular components and it *may be possible to identify agents that can at the same time increase the speed of orthodontic tooth movement while reducing pain*. Recent studies have indicated for example that the transient receptor potential (TRP) vanilloid 1 receptor (TRPV1), a key receptor in pain sensing, is also is expressed in osteoclasts (Rossi et al., 2009; Rossi et al., 2011). TRPV1 is the receptor for capsaicin, the ingredient in red chili peppers that produces burning sensations (Caterina, 2007). Capsaicin and other TRPV1 agonists have been shown to stimulate osteoclast formation (Rossi et al., 2009). From this it is plausible that a single agent, an appropriate agonist of TRPV1, may be able to both relieve orthodontic pain and significantly reduce the time required for orthodontic procedures. Capsaicin is already a FDA-approved treatment for clinical pain and a number of studies have indicated that it is

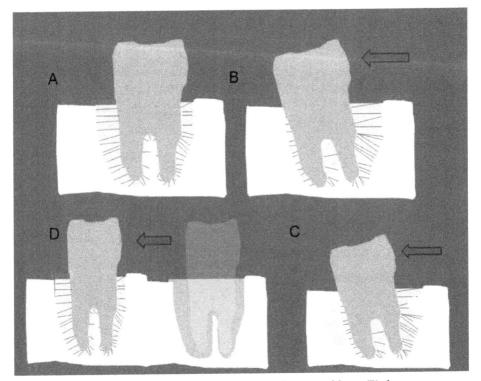

Fig. 1. Orthodontic tooth movement initiates with application of force (B) that compresses the PDL on the pressure side of the tooth, or stretches the periodontal ligament on the tension side. This leads to resorption on the pressure side and bone formation on the tension side (C) which accommodates the repositioning of the tooth (D). Goals of manipulation of tooth movement with bioactive agents include increasing the rate of tooth movement, reducing pain, and preventing relapse

effective in the reduction of pain measures for subjects suffering from arthritis, post-herpetic and diabetic neuropathies (Peikert et al., 1991; McCarthy and McCarty, 1992; Tandan et al., 1992; Watson et al., 1993; Caterina, 2007). As such, an adapted approach might be feasible in the clinic using capsaicin, or other agonists of TRPV1, to easily and safely facilitate the goal of improving orthodontic outcomes.

In summary, opportunities exist for improving orthodontic treatment by enhancing orthodontic tooth movement, preventing relapse, and reducing pain associated with orthodontic procedures (Figure 1). Recent advances in understanding neuromodulation of bone remodeling present new means to affect all of these parameters, perhaps by using the same therapeutic molecule. To examine this in greater detail we will first briefly consider the essential elements of the regulation of bone remodeling, then examine connections between bone cells and neurons.

2. Bone remodeling

Bone remodeling can be thought of simply as a dialog between two cell types, osteoclasts and osteoblasts (Figure 2)(Martin et al., 2009). Osteoclasts are cells of the hematopoetic lineage that are specialized for bone resorption (Teitelbaum, 2007). Osteoblasts are mesenchymal and are specialized for bone formation (Askmyr et al., 2009). Although this is an oversimplification, for example T-cell are known to directly stimulate osteoclast formation and bone resorption (Weitzmann and Pacifici, 2005), and osteocytes are primary regulators of osteoblast bone formation (Winkler et al., 2003; Moester et al., 2010), it is clear

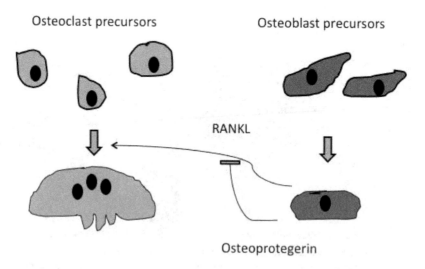

Fig. 2. RANKL produced by osteoblasts stimulates osteoclast formation and osteoclast bone resorption. Osteoprotengerin is also produced by osteoblasts and serves as a competitive inhibitor of RANKL. The humanized monoclonal antibody, denosumab, functions like osteoprotegerin.

that a major element of the regulation of bone remodeling is through expression by osteoblasts of RANKL. This stimulates its receptor, RANK, present on the surface of osteoclast precursors and osteoclasts, which induces osteoclast differentiation, survival and bone resorptive activity (Burgess et al., 1999; Kong et al., 1999). Osteoprotegerin, also produced by osteoblasts, serves as a competitive inhibitor of RANKL and by doing so reduces bone resorption (Hofbauer et al., 2004). Neural regulation of bone remodeling must occur within the constraints of this regulatory system.

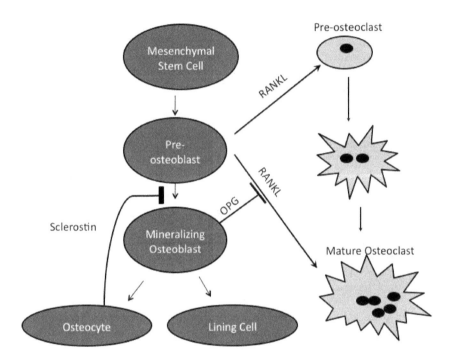

Fig. 3. Sclerostin is thought to inhibit differentiation of osteoblasts from a stage where they promote osteoclastic bone resorption to a stage where they form bone.

RANKL is a tumor necrosis factor (TNF)-related type II transmembrane protein expressed by osteoblasts, T-cells and a few other cell types (Xing et al., 2005). There was great excitement in the bone field in the late 1990s with the demonstration that RANKL was the long sought osteoclast differentiation factor (Lacey et al., 1998). Since the initial reports, this basic finding has been supported by a host of studies (Xing et al., 2005). RANKL binds its receptor RANK to stimulate osteoclast formation and activity. It also binds OPG, which resembles RANK but lacks a transmembrane domain, and serves as a soluble competitive inhibitor. Overwhelming evidence indicates the vital importance of this triad in bone remodeling and has led to the paradigm shown in Figure 2. With the discovery of RANKL came efforts to utilize inhibitors of RANKL in the development of pharmaceutical agents that inhibit osteoclast activity. Recently an anti-RANKL antibody-based pharmaceutical

(Denosumab) was generated by Amgen and approved as an anti-osteoporotic agent (Trade name Prolia) and for bone cancer (Xgeva) (Lewiecki, 2010; Castellano et al., 2011; Baron et al., 2011).

Sclerostin has recently been identified as a vital regulator of bone formation (Moester et al., 2010). Sclerostin is a controller of the Wnt-signaling pathway, which is crucial for modulating bone remodeling (Baron et al., 2006; Kubota et al., 2009). Sclerostin is thought to block the transition of osteoblasts from a step along their differentiation pathway where they produce RANKL, but do not form bone, to a point where they do not produce RANKL (or produce more osteoprotegerin) and do form bone (Figure 3)(Paszty et al., 2010). Thus higher levels of sclerostin will favor bone resorption and lower levels will favor bone formation. Taking advantage of this paradigm, efforts are underway to transition a humanized monoclonal antibody inhibitor of sclerostin to the clinic for the treatment of osteoporosis (Lewiecki, 2011). Sclerostin is one of several molecules that influence osteoblast activity by regulating the Wnt-signaling pathway (Baron et al., 2006).

3. Central control of bone remodeling

During the past decade evidence has accumulated that has shown that levels of bone remodeling and final bone structure is regulated in the central nervous system (Elefteriou, 2008; Wong et al., 2008; Karsenty and Oury, 2010). Three different mechanisms will be discussed in some detail, regulation through leptin signaling, neuropeptide Y and cannibanoid receptors. It is postulated that central regulation of bone remodeling represents a link with bone remodeling and energy metabolism (Karsenty and Oury, 2010). Leptin release by the hypothalamus for example has been shown to regulate both bone remodeling and insulin secretion (Baldock et al., 2002; Takeda, 2008; Kalra et al., 2009; Confavreux et al., 2009; Baldock et al., 2009; Qin et al., 2010; Zengin et al., 2010). Leptin is a 16 kD adipose-derived protein hormone, which plays a key role in regulating energy intake and expenditure. It has a major role in controlling appetite and metabolism.

Evidence suggests that leptin-regulated neural pathways control both bone formation and bone resorption. Mice lacking the gene encoding leptin (ob/ob) are obese and have higher bone mass than normal and higher rates of bone remodeling (Elefteriou et al., 2005). Intracerebroventricular infusion of leptin into the mice, under conditions where little or no leptin leaked into general circulation, led to normalization of both rates of bone remodeling and bone mass (Elefteriou et al., 2005). This strongly supported the idea that leptin regulates bone remodeling through a central relay, and this mode of regulation is vitally important in maintaining bone (Kalra et al., 2009; Karsenty and Oury, 2010).

The leptin receptor is expressed on three types of hypothalamic neurons, although its expression in the brain is not restricted to hypothalamic neurons (Karsenty and Ducy, 2006; Kalra et al., 2009). The three neurons in the hypothalamus are the arcuate nucleus, the ventromedical hypothalamic nucleus, and paraventricular nuclei. Lesioning of the arcuate nucleus using two independent strategies did not affect bone mass directly, or alter the ability of infusion of leptin to affect bone mass (Takeda and Karsenty, 2008). In contrast, lesioning ventromedical hypothalamic nuclei neurons in wild type animals resulted in a high bone mass/high bone turnover phenotype similar to that observe in the ob/ob mice. Infusion of leptin failed to normalize the bone phenotype in either lesioned wild type mice or the ob/ob mice (Guidobono et al., 2006). Taken together, these data suggested that the ventromedical hypothalamic nucleus neurons are required for leptin-dependent central regulation of bone remodeling.

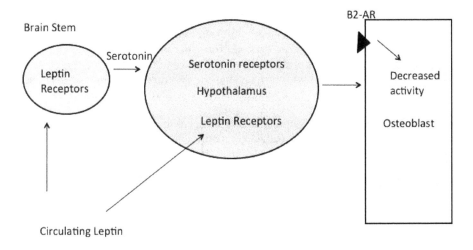

Fig. 4. Leptin stimulates receptors in the brain stem and hypothalamus leading to stimulation of β2 adrenergic receptors in osteoblasts which decrease the activity of osteoblasts

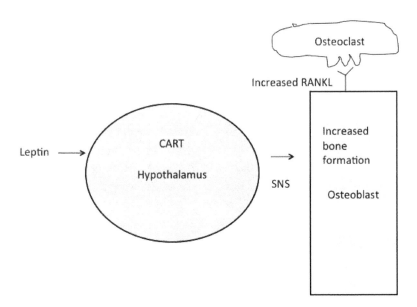

Fig. 5. Leptin stimulates cocaine- and amphetamine- regulated transcript expression which acting through the sympathetic nervous system to stimulate both increased bone formation by osteoblasts and increased resorption by osteoclasts

How then is this regulation mediated? One route is through dopamine β-hydroxylase, an enzyme required for the production of norepinepherine and epinephrine (Figure 4) (Yadav and Karsenty, 2009; Yadav et al., 2009). Mice lacking dopamine β-hydroxylase have a similar bone phenotype to the *ob/ob* mice, and leptin infusion of these mice failed to normalize bone parameters. Only one adrenergic receptor is expressed in osteoblasts, β2 adrenergic receptor. Mice lacking one or both copies of the β2 adrenergic receptor developed a high bone mass phenotype, and leptin infusion into mice lacking the β2 adrenergic receptor decreased fat mass but did not normalize the bone parameters (Yadav and Karsenty, 2009; Yadav et al., 2009).

Another mechanism by which leptin mediates bone remodeling is via the cocaine- and amphetamine- regulated transcript (CART), a neuropeptide precursor protein (Figure 5) (Elefteriou et al., 2005). The level of CART expression in the hypothalamus and peripheral organs including the pancreas and adrenal glands is tied to levels of leptin. Simply, CART expression is stimulated by leptin, and osteoclastic resorption decreases in relation to the amount of CART expressed. This action of CART is mediated through osteoblasts; CART represses RANKL expression of osteoblasts and thus reduces osteoclast formation and bone resorption (Elefteriou et al., 2005).

Neuromedin U is a neuropeptide expressed in hypothalamic neurons and in the small intestine has also been also been implicated as a component of the leptin regulatory pathway (Figure 6) (Sato et al., 2007). Although its receptor is not detected in bone cells, knockout of neuromendin U leads to a high bone mass phenotype. Treatment of leptin deficient mice with neurmedin U resulted in partial rescue of the high bone mass pheneotype suggesting that neuromedin U is downstream of leptin in the bone remodeling regulatory pathway.

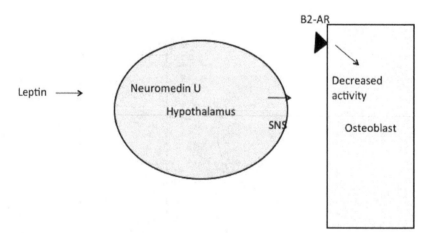

Fig. 6. Leptin also signals through the hypothalamus using a pathway involving neuromedin U and the sympathetic nervous system leading to stimulation of β2 adrenergic receptor which decreases bone formation

Taken together this suggested that leptin regulates bone remodeling through several pathways. Although caution must be exercised in translating these results to humans, they suggest a number of ramifications for humans with respect to orthodontic procedures. First, alterations in elements of this signaling pathway, for example single nucleotide polymorphisms (SNPs) in one or more the genes encoding elements of the pathway may have consequences for the general rate and efficacy of orthodontic procedures in an individual. For example, an SNP in β2 adrenergic receptor that increases signaling from the receptor may be associated with higher than normal bone mineral density, and increased rates of tooth movement.

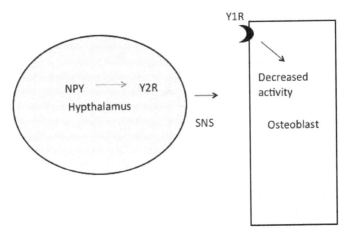

Fig. 7. Neuropeptide Y signals through Y2R receptors in the hypothalamus and Y1R receptors in osteoblasts to decrease osteoblast activity

Secondly, direct local stimulation of osteoblasts in the alveolar bone associated with specific teeth with β2 adrenergic receptor agonists might both enhance rates of tooth movement and increase the speed of bone formation at the tension side of the tooth, perhaps reducing the tendency to relapse. However, care would have to be taken in manipulating these pathways because of the associations of the adrenergic systems with cardiovascular diseases (Saini-Chohan and Hatch, 2009). In addition, a recent study indicated that SNPs in the β2 adrenergic receptor are associated with heterotypic ossification, which is associated with higher rates of fractures. Moreover, recent studies of bisphosphonate-associated oral osteonecrosis suggests that the condition is actually osteosclerosis, and may result from disorganization of normal bone remodeling rather than blocking of the process (Chiu et al., 2010; Treister et al., 2010). *While perturbation in normal bone remodeling on the surface may have favorable outcomes, great care must be taken due to the complexity of bone formation and remodeling which can lead to unexpected adverse consequences.*

Neuropeptide Y, a neurotransmitter that is widely expressed in both central and peripheral nervous systems, has been shown to regulate bone remodeling (Baldock et al., 2007; Baldock et al., 2009)(Figure 7). Knockout mice of either the neuropeptide Y1 or Y2 receptors yielded a high bone mass phenotype with enhanced osteoblast activity (Baldock et al., 2009). Neuropeptide Y receptors are, like the leptin receptor, expressed by cells of the hypothalamus. Knockout of Y2 in the hypothalamus is sufficient to induce a high bone density phenotype. However, knockout of Y1 in the hypothalamus did not alter bone homeostasis (Baldock et al., 2002; Baldock et al., 2007).

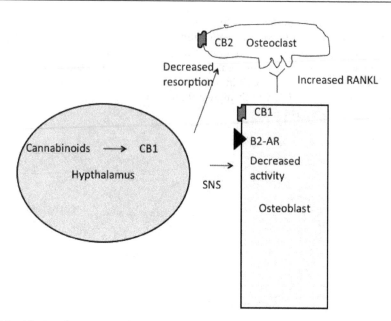

Fig. 8. Cannabinoid stimulate a central response that leads to decreased bone formation. The CB2 receptor of osteoclasts reduces osteoclast activity, but CB1 stimulation increases expression of RANKL which is pro-stimulatory

Recently, the Y1 receptor was knocked out specifically in osteoblasts using a Cre/Lox system (Baldock et al., 2007). It was shown that osteoblast specific knockout of Y1 was sufficient to increase bone mass and enhance bone remodeling. These data indicated that neuropeptide Y signaling could have a role in both central and local neural control of bone remodeling.

Neuropeptide Y signaling has been linked to food intake and like leptin, there are links between neuropeptide Y signaling and obesity (Munoz and Argente, 2002; Feletou and Levens, 2005). Neuropeptide Y receptors are found on pre- and post-synaptic neurons. Presumably activation of the receptors is tied to behavioral changes leading to alterations in food consumption. Whether it is possible to take advantage of neuropeptide Y signaling to influence bone remodeling associated with orthodontic applications is not clear, but most likely, means would have to be devised to deliver agonists locally.

A third route by which bone remodeling can be regulated centrally in through endocannabinoid signaling, which has been shown modulate bone remodeling through central and peripheral cannabinoid receptors(Davenport, 2005; Rossi et al., 2009) (Figure 8). Cannabinoid receptors are a class of G protein coupled membrane receptors. The cannabinoid receptors CB1 and CB2 play a key role in the maintenance of bone mass and are expressed on osteoblasts, osteoclasts and osteocytes. Deficiency in the hypothalamic receptor CB1 in mice has been shown to accelerate age-dependent osteoporosis. Agonists of CB2 reduce bone loss after ovariectomy in rodent models while increasing the thickness of the cortical bone. This makes CB2 a potential target for agents designed to modulate bone remodeling.

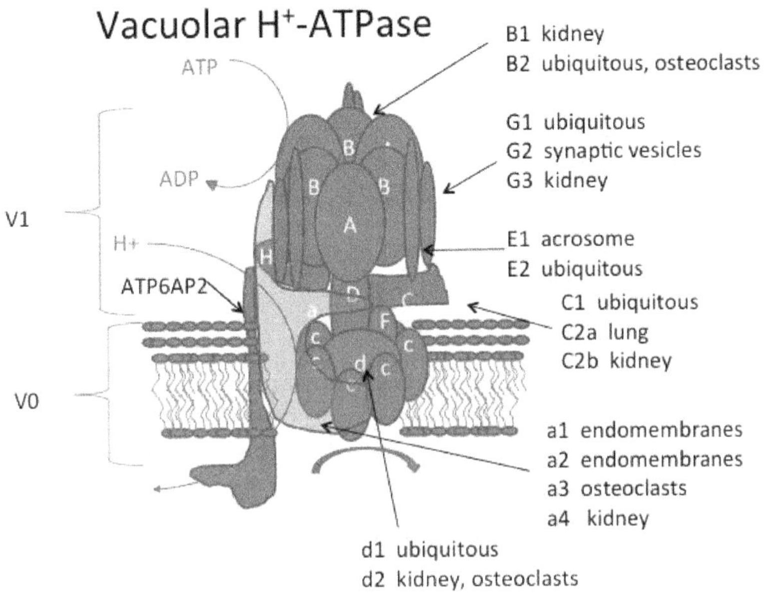

Fig. 9. V-ATPases are ubiquitously-expressed and are composed of many subunits. Some subunits are present in multiple isoforms. Osteoclasts, for example, contain the "housekeeping" isoforms of subunit a (a1, and a2) and the also express the a3 subunit which is required for bone resorption. ATP6AP2 (the prorenein receptor) links bone resorption to rennin/angiotensin signalling.

4. Common molecular features shared by neurons and bone cells

4.1 Specialized machinery for acidification

Evidence has emerged that osteoclasts share a number of molecular features with neural cells. These include the specialized use of vacuolar H^+-ATPase (V-ATPase), chloride channel protein 7 (CLC-7), which work in coordination in order to properly acidify compartments (Schaller et al., 2005; Hinton et al., 2009).

The V-ATPase is a multisubunit enzyme (11-13 subunits) that is expressed in all cells and is required for "housekeeping" acidification of vesicular compartments including lysosomes, late endosomes, compartments of uncoupling receptor and ligand, elements of the golgi, and phagosomes (Hinton et al., 2009). Certain specialized cell types express both the housekeeping subset of V-ATPases, and in addition, an additional subset that is involved in the specialized function of the cell type (Figure 9).

Osteoclasts, which are specialized to resorb bone, are a clear and well-characterized example of a cell type that uses V-ATPases for a specialized function (Blair et al., 1989; Holliday et al., 2005). Osteoclasts express normal housekeeping V-ATPases (Toyomura et al., 2003). In addition, they express a large subset that is destined for the plasma membrane of resorbing cells. When an osteoclast contacts activation signals associated with the bone surface, the specialized subset of V-ATPases is transported to a subdomain of the plasma membrane called the ruffled plasma membrane or ruffled border (Blair et al., 1989). These V-ATPases then use ATP hydrolysis to pump protons against an electrochemical gradient to acidify an extracellular resorption compartment (Figure 10).

Different subsets of V-ATPases are distinguished by isoforms of particular subunits. Some subunits are present in only a single form and are present in all V-ATPases no matter what their function. Others have multiple isoforms that are derived from different genes. For example, there are four isoforms of the a subunit (a1-a4). Subunits a1 and a2 are found in the housekeeping V-ATPases. The a3-subunit has been identified at high levels in osteoclasts, pancreatic beta cells, kidney epithelial cells and microglia (Li et al., 1999; Smith et al., 2001; Sun-Wada et al., 2006; Serrano et al., 2009). The a4 subunit is restricted to epithelial cells of the kidney (Stover et al., 2002).

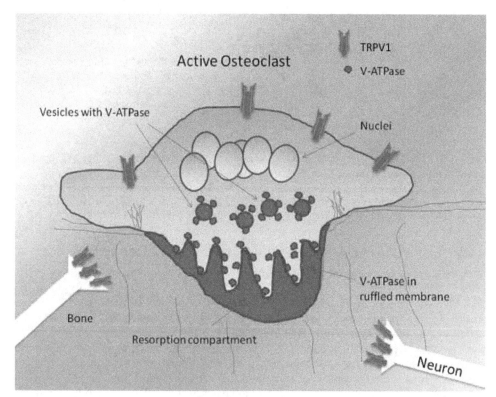

Fig. 10. Osteoclasts insert V-ATPases into the plasma membrane is a region known as the ruffled border. V-ATPases pump protons into the resorption compartment lowering the pH, which is crucial for bone resorption. TRPV1 is expressed on both osteoclasts, where agonists are proresorptive, and on neurons, where agonists reduce pain. This makes it possible that a single therapeutic agent can both increase the rate of tooth movement (which requires increased osteoclastic resorption) and reduce pain associated with orthodontic procedures.

Like osteoclasts, neurons also express subsets of V-ATPases that are utilized for specialized purposes (Moriyama et al., 1992). Neurons are thought to utilize V-ATPases to generate a driving force to power loading synaptic vesicles with neurotransmitters. In addition, there is considerable evidence that a subunit is intimately involved in mediating the fusion of synaptic vesicles with the plasma membrane to allow dumping of neurotransmitters into the synaptic cleft (Hiesinger et al., 2005; Di et al., 2010).

Among the most exciting recent findings was the demonstration that a V-ATPase accessory protein, the pro-renin receptor (PRR, also known as ATP6AP2) forms a vital scaffold between V-ATPase and the Wnt-signaling pathway (Cruciat et al., 2010). Without PRR, mineralization was blocked in a mouse model. Whether PRR is also found in osteoclasts is not known, and whether the recent demonstration that PRR is found in the hypothalamus suggests that it may be another molecule by which central regulation of bone remodeling might occur remains to be explored (Takahashi et al., 2010). In this case, the primary known function of PRR is its involvement in renin-angiotensin signaling which is related to blood pressure and cardiac activity (Nguyen, 2011).

Along with sharing specialized functions of V-ATPases, both neurons and osteoclasts require the voltage–gated chloride channel CLC-7. This channel is thought to open to reduce voltage across membranes produced by the activity of electrogenic V-ATPases. Mutations in CLC-7 lead to both osteopetrosis and neurodegeneration (Kornak et al., 2001; Kasper et al., 2005)

4.2 Sensing receptors shared by neurons and osteoclasts

Both bone remodeling and sensory pain pathways share common inflammatory mediators, including TNF-α, prostaglandins, interleukins, and vasoactive neuropeptides (e.g., substance P), to name a few. Again, specifically targeting the intersection of these pathways may provide unique opportunities for development of innovative therapies related to bone disorders and specifically OTM. The transient receptor potential (TRP) channels is a class of receptors that are involved in sensory and pain processing. For example, The TRP vanilloid 1 receptor (**TRPV1**) is found primarily on neuronal c- and a-δ fiber nociceptors that are responsible for thermal/burning pain. TRPV1 is also a major transducer of inflammatory pain, especially under acidic conditions. Recent work demonstrated that TRPV1 is expressed in human **osteoclasts**, indicating that TRPV1 may promote bone resorption (Rossi et al., 2009; Rossi et al., 2011). Previous work with ultrapotent TRPV1 agonists such as resiniferatoxin (RTX) indicates that inflammatory pain can be eliminated (Neubert, et al. 2008). TRPV1 is activated in response to lowered pH, which is an important regulator of local bone resorption. TRPV1 is expressed on osteoclasts and agonists of TRPV1, capsaicin and resinoferotoxin (RTX), stimulate osteoclast differentiation at concentrations where neuronal pain sensors are not inactivated (Rossi et al., 2009; Rossi et al., 2011). Interestingly, agonists of TRPV1 induce overexpression of the cannabinoid receptor CB2 (Rossi et al., 2009; Rossi et al., 2011). The TRPV1 inhibitor capsazepine was also shown to inhibit both osteoclast and osteoblast differentiation (Idris et al., 2010). Together, this makes TRPV1 a potential integrator between the central nervous system and bone which may be involved in orchestrating both local bone remodeling changes in response to pH and possibly orthodontic force, and augmenting central modulation of bone remodeling. These data suggest that well documented agonists and antagonists of TRPV1 may prove to be ideal agents for manipulation of OTM in ways by which orthodontic practice may be improved. Increased understanding of OTM can also provide insight into mechanisms of bone biology.

Interestingly, agonists of TRPV1 induce overexpression of the cannabinoid receptor CB2 (Rossi et al., 2009; Rossi et al., 2011). Increased understanding of OTM can provide insight into mechanisms of bone biology. For example, this knowledge may have direct implications for the use of TRPV1 agonists in the treatment of pain and bone destruction associated with bone cancer [10] (Figure 10).

5. Summary

Biological manipulation to improve orthodontic procedures is in its infancy, but it appears possible to both improve the speed and efficacy of tooth movement, and to reduce associated discomfort. Proof-in-principle experiments have been performed in animal models but translation to the clinic will require greater understanding of the processes involved. Recent studies uncovering mechanisms by which bone remodeling is controlled by central mechanisms and demonstrating that osteoclasts and neurons share regulatory molecules, although they are used for different purposes, open new avenues for understanding and manipulating orthodontic tooth movement and perhaps simultaneously reducing the discomfort associated with the procedures.

6. References

Wise, G. E. and King, G. J. (2008). Mechanisms of tooth eruption and orthodontic tooth movement. *J. Dent. Res.* 87, 414-434.

Krishnan, V. and Davidovitch, Z. (2006). Cellular, molecular, and tissue-level reactions to orthodontic force. *Am. J. Orthod. Dentofacial Orthop.* 129, 469-32.

Kanzaki, H., Chiba, M., Arai, K., Takahashi, I., Haruyama, N., Nishimura, M. and Mitani, H. (2006). Local RANKL gene transfer to the periodontal tissue accelerates orthodontic tooth movement. *Gene Ther.* 13, 678-685.

Hofbauer, L. C. and Heufelder, A. E. (2001). Role of receptor activator of nuclear factor-kappaB ligand and osteoprotegerin in bone cell biology. *J. Mol. Med.* 79, 243-253.

Dunn, M. D., Park, C. H., Kostenuik, P. J., Kapila, S. and Giannobile, W. V. (2007). Local delivery of osteoprotegerin inhibits mechanically mediated bone modeling in orthodontic tooth movement. *Bone* 41, 446-455.

Kanzaki, H., Chiba, M., Takahashi, I., Haruyama, N., Nishimura, M. and Mitani, H. (2004). Local OPG gene transfer to periodontal tissue inhibits orthodontic tooth movement. *Journal of Dental Research* 83, 920-925.

Dolce, C., Vakani, A., Archer, L., Morris-Wiman, J. A. and Holliday, L. S. (2003). Effects of echistatin and an RGD peptide on orthodontic tooth movement. *Journal of Dental Research* 82, 682-686.

Holliday, L. S., Vakani, A., Archer, L. and Dolce, C. (2003). Effects of matrix metalloproteinase inhibitors on bone resorption and orthodontic tooth movement. *J. Dent. Res.* 82, 687-691.

Moester, M. J., Papapoulos, S. E., Lowik, C. W. and Van Bezooijen, R. L. (2010). Sclerostin: current knowledge and future perspectives. *Calcif. Tissue Int.* 87, 99-107.

Paszty, C., Turner, C. H. and Robinson, M. K. (2010). Sclerostin: a gem from the genome leads to bone-building antibodies. *J. Bone Miner. Res.* 25, 1897-1904.

Kehoe, M. J., Cohen, S. M., Zarrinnia, K. and Cowan, A. (1996). The effect of acetaminophen, ibuprofen, and misoprostol on prostaglandin E2 synthesis and the degree and rate of orthodontic tooth movement. *Angle Orthod.* 66, 339-349.

Simmons, K. E. and Brandt, M. (1992). Control of orthodontic pain. *J. Indiana Dent. Assoc.* 71, 8-10.

Walker, J. B. and Buring, S. M. (2001). NSAID impairment of orthodontic tooth movement. *Ann. Pharmacother.* 35, 113-115.

Bergius, M., Kiliaridis, S. and Berggren, U. (2000). Pain in orthodontics. A review and discussion of the literature. *J. Orofac. Orthop.* 61, 125-137.

Eversole, L. R. (2006). Evidence-based practice of oral pathology and oral medicine. *J. Calif. Dent. Assoc.* 34, 448-454.

Giannopoulou, C., Dudic, A. and Kiliaridis, S. (2006). Pain discomfort and crevicular fluid changes induced by orthodontic elastic separators in children. *J. Pain* 7, 367-376.

Rossi, F., Siniscalco, D., Luongo, L., De, P. L., Bellini, G., Petrosino, S., Torella, M., Santoro, C., Nobili, B., Perrotta, S. et al. (2009). The endovanilloid/endocannabinoid system in human osteoclasts: possible involvement in bone formation and resorption. *Bone* 44, 476-484.

Rossi, F., Bellini, G., Luongo, L., Torella, M., Mancusi, S., De, P. L., Petrosino, S., Siniscalco, D., Orlando, P., Scafuro, M. et al. (2011). The endovanilloid/endocannabinoid system: A new potential target for osteoporosis therapy. *Bone.*

Caterina, M. J. (2007). Transient receptor potential ion channels as participants in thermosensation and thermoregulation. *Am. J. Physiol Regul. Integr. Comp Physiol* 292, R64-R76.

McCarthy, G. M. and McCarty, D. J. (1992). Effect of topical capsaicin in the therapy of painful osteoarthritis of the hands. *J. Rheumatol.* 19, 604-607.

Peikert, A., Hentrich, M. and Ochs, G. (1991). Topical 0.025% capsaicin in chronic post-herpetic neuralgia: efficacy, predictors of response and long-term course. *J. Neurol.* 238, 452-456.

Tandan, R., Lewis, G. A., Krusinski, P. B., Badger, G. B. and Fries, T. J. (1992). Topical capsaicin in painful diabetic neuropathy. Controlled study with long-term follow-up. *Diabetes Care* 15, 8-14.

Watson, C. P., Tyler, K. L., Bickers, D. R., Millikan, L. E., Smith, S. and Coleman, E. (1993). A randomized vehicle-controlled trial of topical capsaicin in the treatment of postherpetic neuralgia. *Clin. Ther.* 15, 510-526.

Martin, T., Gooi, J. H. and Sims, N. A. (2009). Molecular mechanisms in coupling of bone formation to resorption. *Crit Rev. Eukaryot. Gene Expr.* 19, 73-88.

Teitelbaum, S. L. (2007). Osteoclasts: what do they do and how do they do it? *Am. J. Pathol.* 170, 427-435.

Askmyr, M., Sims, N. A., Martin, T. J. and Purton, L. E. (2009). What is the true nature of the osteoblastic hematopoietic stem cell niche? *Trends Endocrinol. Metab* 20, 303-309.

Weitzmann, M. N. and Pacifici, R. (2005). The role of T lymphocytes in bone metabolism. *Immunological Reviews* 208, 154-168.

Winkler, D. G., Sutherland, M. K., Geoghegan, J. C., Yu, C., Hayes, T., Skonier, J. E., Shpektor, D., Jonas, M., Kovacevich, B. R., Staehling-Hampton, K. et al. (2003). Osteocyte control of bone formation via sclerostin, a novel BMP antagonist. *EMBO J.* 22, 6267-6276.

Burgess, T. L., Qian, Y., Kaufman, S., Ring, B. D., Van, G., Capparelli, C., Kelley, M., Hsu, H., Boyle, W. J., Dunstan, C. R. et al. (1999). The ligand for osteoprotegerin (OPGL) directly activates mature osteoclasts. *J. Cell Biol.* 145, 527-538.

Kong, Y. Y., Yoshida, H., Sarosi, I., Tan, H. L., Timms, E., Capparelli, C., Morony, S., Oliveira-dos-Santos, A. J., Van, G., Itie, A. et al. (1999). OPGL is a key regulator of osteoclastogenesis, lymphocyte development and lymph-node organogenesis. *Nature* 397, 315-323.

Hofbauer, L. C., Kuhne, C. A. and Viereck, V. (2004). The OPG/RANKL/RANK system in metabolic bone diseases. *J. Musculoskelet. Neuronal. Interact.* 4, 268-275.

Xing, L. P., Schwarz, E. M. and Boyce, B. F. (2005). Osteoclast precursors, RANKL/RANK, and immunology. *Immunological Reviews* 208, 19-29.

Lacey, D. L., Timms, E., Tan, H. L., Kelley, M. J., Dunstan, C. R., Burgess, T., Elliott, R., Colombero, A., Elliott, G., Scully, S. et al. (1998). Osteoprotegerin ligand is a cytokine that regulates osteoclast differentiation and activation. *Cell* 93, 165-176.

Lewiecki, E. M. (2010). Denosumab--an emerging treatment for postmenopausal osteoporosis. *Expert. Opin. Biol. Ther.* 10, 467-476.

Baron, R., Ferrari, S. and Russell, R. G. (2011). Denosumab and bisphosphonates: Different mechanisms of action and effects. *Bone* 48, 677-692.

Castellano, D., Sepulveda, J. M., Garcia-Escobar, I., Rodriguez-Antolin, A., Sundlov, A. and Cortes-Funes, H. (2011). The role of RANK-ligand inhibition in cancer: the story of denosumab. *Oncologist.* 16, 136-145.

Baron, R., Rawadi, G. and Roman-Roman, S. (2006). Wnt signaling: a key regulator of bone mass. *Curr. Top. Dev. Biol.* 76, 103-127.

Kubota, T., Michigami, T. and Ozono, K. (2009). Wnt signaling in bone metabolism. *J. Bone Miner. Metab* 27, 265-271.

Lewiecki, E. M. (2011). Sclerostin monoclonal antibody therapy with AMG 785: a potential treatment for osteoporosis. *Expert. Opin. Biol. Ther.* 11, 117-127.

Elefteriou, F. (2008). Regulation of bone remodeling by the central and peripheral nervous system. *Arch. Biochem. Biophys.* 473, 231-236.

Karsenty, G. and Oury, F. (2010). The central regulation of bone mass, the first link between bone remodeling and energy metabolism. *J. Clin. Endocrinol. Metab* 95, 4795-4801.

Wong, I. P., Zengin, A., Herzog, H. and Baldock, P. A. (2008). Central regulation of bone mass. *Semin. Cell Dev. Biol.* 19, 452-458.

Confavreux, C. B., Levine, R. L. and Karsenty, G. (2009). A paradigm of integrative physiology, the crosstalk between bone and energy metabolisms. *Mol. Cell Endocrinol.* 310, 21-29.

Kalra, S. P., Dube, M. G. and Iwaniec, U. T. (2009). Leptin increases osteoblast-specific osteocalcin release through a hypothalamic relay. *Peptides* 30, 967-973.

Baldock, P. A., Sainsbury, A., Couzens, M., Enriquez, R. F., Thomas, G. P., Gardiner, E. M. and Herzog, H. (2002). Hypothalamic Y2 receptors regulate bone formation. *J. Clin. Invest* 109, 915-921.

Baldock, P. A., Lee, N. J., Driessler, F., Lin, S., Allison, S., Stehrer, B., Lin, E. J., Zhang, L., Enriquez, R. F., Wong, I. P. et al. (2009). Neuropeptide Y knockout mice reveal a central role of NPY in the coordination of bone mass to body weight. *PLoS. ONE.* 4, e8415.

Qin, W., Bauman, W. A. and Cardozo, C. P. (2010). Evolving concepts in neurogenic osteoporosis. *Curr. Osteoporos. Rep.* 8, 212-218.

Takeda, S. (2008). Central control of bone remodelling. *J. Neuroendocrinol.* 20, 802-807.

Zengin, A., Zhang, L., Herzog, H., Baldock, P. A. and Sainsbury, A. (2010). Neuropeptide Y and sex hormone interactions in humoral and neuronal regulation of bone and fat. *Trends Endocrinol. Metab* 21, 411-418.

Elefteriou, F., Ahn, J. D., Takeda, S., Starbuck, M., Yang, X., Liu, X., Kondo, H., Richards, W. G., Bannon, T. W., Noda, M. et al. (2005). Leptin regulation of bone resorption by the sympathetic nervous system and CART. *Nature* 434, 514-520.

Karsenty, G. and Ducy, P. (2006). The hypothalamic control of bone mass, implication for the treatment of osteoporosis. *Ann. Endocrinol. (Paris)* 67, 123.

Takeda, S. and Karsenty, G. (2008). Molecular bases of the sympathetic regulation of bone mass. *Bone* 42, 837-840.

Guidobono, F., Pagani, F., Sibilia, V., Netti, C., Lattuada, N., Rapetti, D., Mrak, E., Villa, I., Cavani, F., Bertoni, L. et al. (2006). Different skeletal regional response to continuous brain infusion of leptin in the rat. *Peptides* 27, 1426-1433.

Yadav, V. K. and Karsenty, G. (2009). Leptin-dependent co-regulation of bone and energy metabolism. *Aging (Albany. NY)* 1, 954-956.

Yadav, V. K., Oury, F., Suda, N., Liu, Z. W., Gao, X. B., Confavreux, C., Klemenhagen, K. C., Tanaka, K. F., Gingrich, J. A., Guo, X. E. et al. (2009). A serotonin-dependent mechanism explains the leptin regulation of bone mass, appetite, and energy expenditure. *Cell* 138, 976-989.

Sato, S., Hanada, R., Kimura, A., Abe, T., Matsumoto, T., Iwasaki, M., Inose, H., Ida, T., Mieda, M., Takeuchi, Y. et al. (2007). Central control of bone remodeling by neuromedin U. *Nat. Med.* 13, 1234-1240.

Saini-Chohan, H. K. and Hatch, G. M. (2009). Biological actions and metabolism of currently used pharmacological agents for the treatment of congestive heart failure. *Curr. Drug Metab* 10, 206-219.

Chiu, C. T., Chiang, W. F., Chuang, C. Y. and Chang, S. W. (2010). Resolution of oral bisphosphonate and steroid-related osteonecrosis of the jaw--a serial case analysis. *J. Oral Maxillofac. Surg.* 68, 1055-1063.

Treister, N. S., Friedland, B. and Woo, S. B. (2010). Use of cone-beam computerized tomography for evaluation of bisphosphonate-associated osteonecrosis of the jaws. *Oral Surg. Oral Med. Oral Pathol. Oral Radiol. Endod.* 109, 753-764.

Baldock, P. A., Allison, S. J., Lundberg, P., Lee, N. J., Slack, K., Lin, E. J., Enriquez, R. F., McDonald, M. M., Zhang, L., During, M. J. et al. (2007). Novel role of Y1 receptors in the coordinated regulation of bone and energy homeostasis. *J. Biol. Chem.* 282, 19092-19102.

Feletou, M. and Levens, N. R. (2005). Neuropeptide Y2 receptors as drug targets for the central regulation of body weight. *Curr. Opin. Investig. Drugs* 6, 1002-1011.

Munoz, M. T. and Argente, J. (2002). Anorexia nervosa in female adolescents: endocrine and bone mineral density disturbances. *Eur. J. Endocrinol.* 147, 275-286.

Davenport, R. J. (2005). The skeleton goes to pot. *Sci. Aging Knowledge. Environ.* 2005, nf39.

Hinton, A., Bond, S. and Forgac, M. (2009). V-ATPase functions in normal and disease processes. *Pflugers Arch.* 457, 589-598.

Schaller, S., Henriksen, K., Sorensen, M. G. and Karsdal, M. A. (2005). The role of chloride channels in osteoclasts: ClC-7 as a target for osteoporosis treatment. *Drug News Perspect.* 18, 489-495.

Blair, H. C., Teitelbaum, S. L., Ghiselli, R. and Gluck, S. (1989). Osteoclastic bone resorption by a polarized vacuolar proton pump. *Science* 245, 855-857.

Holliday, L. S., Bubb, M. R., Jiang, J., Hurst, I. R. and Zuo, J. (2005). Interactions between vacuolar H+-ATPases and microfilaments in osteoclasts. *Journal of Bioenergetics and Biomembranes* 37, 419-423.

Toyomura, T., Murata, Y., Yamamoto, A., Oka, T., Sun-Wada, G. H., Wada, Y. and Futai, M. (2003). From Lysosomes to the Plasma Membrane: LOCALIZATION OF VACUOLAR TYPE H+-ATPase WITH THE a3 ISOFORM DURING OSTEOCLAST DIFFERENTIATION. *J. Biol. Chem.* 278, 22023-22030.

Li, Y. P., Chen, W., Liang, Y., Li, E. and Stashenko, P. (1999). Atp6i-deficient mice exhibit severe osteopetrosis due to loss of osteoclast-mediated extracellular acidification. *Nat. Genet.* 23, 447-451.

Sun-Wada, G. H., Toyomura, T., Murata, Y., Yamamoto, A., Futai, M. and Wada, Y. (2006). The a3 isoform of V-ATPase regulates insulin secretion from pancreatic beta-cells. *J. Cell Sci.* 119, 4531-4540.

Smith, A. N., Finberg, K. E., Wagner, C. A., Lifton, R. P., Devonald, M. A., Su, Y. and Karet, F. E. (2001). Molecular cloning and characterization of Atp6n1b: a novel fourth murine vacuolar H+-ATPase a-subunit gene. *J. Biol. Chem.* 276, 42382-42388.

Serrano, E. M., Ricofort, R. D., Zuo, J., Ochotny, N., Manolson, M. F. and Holliday, L. S. (2009). Regulation of vacuolar H(+)-ATPase in microglia by RANKL. *Biochem. Biophys. Res. Commun.* 389, 193-197.

Stover, E. H., Borthwick, K. J., Bavalia, C., Eady, N., Fritz, D. M., Rungroj, N., Giersch, A. B., Morton, C. C., Axon, P. R., Akil, I. et al. (2002). Novel ATP6V1B1 and ATP6V0A4 mutations in autosomal recessive distal renal tubular acidosis with new evidence for hearing loss. *J. Med. Genet.* 39, 796-803.

Moriyama, Y., Maeda, M. and Futai, M. (1992). The role of V-ATPase in neuronal and endocrine systems. *J. Exp. Biol.* 172, 171-178.

Neubert JK, Mannes AJ, Karai LJ, Jenkins AC, Zawatski L, Abu-Asab M, Iadarola MJ. (2008). Perineural resiniferatoxin selectively inhibits inflammatory hyperalgesia. Mol Pain. 2008 Jan 16;4:3.

Di, G. J., Boudkkazi, S., Mochida, S., Bialowas, A., Samari, N., Leveque, C., Youssouf, F., Brechet, A., Iborra, C., Maulet, Y. et al. (2010). V-ATPase membrane sector associates with synaptobrevin to modulate neurotransmitter release. *Neuron 67*, 268-279.

Hiesinger, P. R., Fayyazuddin, A., Mehta, S. Q., Rosenmund, T., Schulze, K. L., Zhai, R. G., Verstreken, P., Cao, Y., Zhou, Y., Kunz, J. et al. (2005). The v-ATPase V-0 subunit a1 is required for a late step in synaptic vesicle exocytosis in Drosophila. *Cell* 121, 607-620.

Cruciat, C. M., Ohkawara, B., Acebron, S. P., Karaulanov, E., Reinhard, C., Ingelfinger, D., Boutros, M. and Niehrs, C. (2010). Requirement of prorenin receptor and vacuolar H+-ATPase-mediated acidification for Wnt signaling. *Science* 327, 459-463.

Takahashi, K., Hiraishi, K., Hirose, T., Kato, I., Yamamoto, H., Shoji, I., Shibasaki, A., Kaneko, K., Satoh, F. and Totsune, K. (2010). Expression of (pro)renin receptor in the human brain and pituitary, and co-localisation with arginine vasopressin and oxytocin in the hypothalamus. *J. Neuroendocrinol.* 22, 453-459.

Nguyen, G. (2011). Renin and Prorenin Receptor in Hypertension: What's New? *Curr. Hypertens. Rep.* 13, 79-85.

Kasper, D., Planells-Cases, R., Fuhrmann, J. C., Scheel, O., Zeitz, O., Ruether, K., Schmitt, A., Poet, M., Steinfeld, R., Schweizer, M. et al. (2005). Loss of the chloride channel ClC-7 leads to lysosomal storage disease and neurodegeneration. *EMBO J.* 24, 1079-1091.

Kornak, U., Kasper, D., Bosl, M. R., Kaiser, E., Schweizer, M., Schulz, A., Friedrich, W., Delling, G. and Jentsch, T. J. (2001). Loss of the ClC-7 chloride channel leads to osteopetrosis in mice and man. *Cell* 104, 205-215.

Idris, A. I., Landao-Bassonga, E. and Ralston, S. H. (2010). The TRPV1 ion channel antagonist capsazepine inhibits osteoclast and osteoblast differentiation in vitro and ovariectomy induced bone loss in vivo. *Bone* 46, 1089-1099.

8

The Artificial Intelligence Approach for Diagnosis, Treatment and Modelling in Orthodontic

Kazem Bahaa[1], Garma Noor[2] and Yousif Yousif[3]
[1]Mechatronics Eng. Dept., Baghdad University,
[2]Orthodontic Dept., Dentistry College, Baghdad University,
[3]Ministry of Higher Education and Scientific Research/ R&D Department,
Baghdad
Iraq

1. Introduction

The discipline, science, and art of orthodontics are concerned with the face and ability to modify its growth. Orthodontists achieve their goals by manipulating the craniofacial skeleton, with particular emphasis on modifying the dentoalveolar region, external orthopedic forces are applied that mirror some techniques used in medical orthopedics. Most treatments, however, focus on modifying the occlusion and controlling dentoalveolar development and abnormal facial growth, thus, enormous amounts of designs and techniques invented in the diagnostic and treatment domains aiming at boolean etiological identification and optimized strategies of solution delivered. A valid problem assessment enables health providers to determine treatment need and priority, and as health care moves toward more stringent financial accountability. the inventory of the computer and its implementation in different medical field was of great interest, this interest are even greater with the artificial intelligence introduction (AI).

The best definition for the phrase "AI" calls for formalization of the term "intelligence". Psychologist and cognitive theorists are of the opinion that intelligence helps in identifying the right piece of knowledge at the appropriate instances of decision making [1,2].The phrase "AI" thus can be defined as the simulation of human intelligence on a machine. Thus, AI alternatively may be stated as a subject dealing with computational models that can think and act rationally [3-7].

The subject of AI spans a wide horizon. It deals with the various kinds of knowledge representation schemes, different techniques of intelligent search, various methods for resolving uncertainty of data and knowledge, diffrent schemes for automated machine learning and many others. Among the application areas of AI, we have Expert systems, Game-playing, and Theorem-proving, Natural language processing, Image recognition, Robotics and many others. This chapter aims at bringing the insight of interest to the conjugation relatively recently happened between orthodontics discipline and AI subject.

2. Introduction to AI

The subject of AI was originated with game-playing and theorem-proving programs and was gradually progressed with theories from a number of parent disciplines. As a young discipline of science, the significance of the topics covered under the subject changes considerably with time. The subject of AI has been enriched with a wide discipline of knowledge from Philosophy, Psychology, Cognitive Science, Computer Science, Mathematics and Engineering. Thus in fig.1, they have been referred to as the parent disciplines of AI.

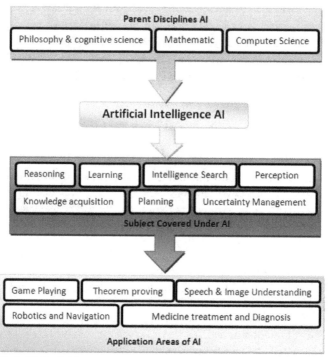

Fig. 1. Parent disciplines of AI

2.1 Artificial neural nets

Neural networks are composed of simple elements operating in parallel. These elements are inspired by biological nervous systems. As in nature, the network function is determined largely by the connections between elements. You can train a neural network to perform a particular function by adjusting the values of the connections (weights) between elements , fig. 2. Commonly neural networks are adjusted, or trained, so that a particular input leads to a specific target output. Such a situation can be shown as follows: there, the network is adjusted, based on a comparison of the output and the target, until the network output matches the target. Typically many such input/target pairs are needed to train a network [7,8]. One type of network sees the nodes as 'artificial neurons'. These are called Artificial Neural Networks (ANNs). Natural neurons receive signals through synapses located on the dendrites or membrane of the neuron. When the signals received are strong enough (surpass a certain threshold), the neuron is activated and emits a signal though the axon. This signal might be sent to another synapse, and might activate other neurons.

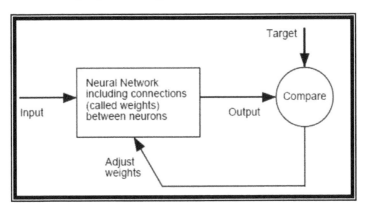

Fig. 2. Basic operation of ANN [9]

An interconnected assembly of simple processing elements, units or nodes, whose functionality is loosely based on the animal brain. The processing ability of the network is stored in the inter unit connection strengths, weights, obtained by a process of adaptation to, or learning from, a set of training patterns.

The benefits of using the neural network can be summarized as follows [10]:

1. Nonlinearity: an artificial neuron can be linear or non-linear a neural netmade up of interconnection of non-linear neurons, is itself non-linear, note that even linear function could be modeled by non-linear neurons, while the inverse can't be done.

2. Input and output mapping: usual learning process of neural network carried out in a popular paradigm of learning called learning with teacher "supervised learning" here modification of synaptic weights of a neural network done by applying set of labeled training samples, each sample consist of a unique input signal and a corresponding desired response. The previous samples could be arranged in different manners so the network constructing an input output mapping for the problem.

3. Adaptively: neural networks have a built in capability to adapt their synaptic to change in the surrounding environment. This could be done by retraining of the model or make the network changes itssynaptic weights in real time and this will be useful for pattern classification, signal processing, and control application.

4. Fault tolerance: a neural network, implemented in hard ware form, has the potential to be inherently fault tolerance, or capable of robust control. For example if a neuron or its connecting links are damaged and due to the nature of distributed information in neural network, this damage little effect on network response.

Neural Network Architecture: A neuron is an information-processing unit that is fundamental to the operation of a neural network. The block diagram of fig. 3 shows the model of a neuron, which forms the basis for designing (artificial) neural network.

The neuronal model of fig. (3) also includes an externally applied bias, denoted by (bk). The bias (bk) has the effect of increasing or lowering the net put of the activation function, depending on whether it is positive or negative, respectively [11], fig 4 shows common types of activation functions.

In mathematical terms:

$$f(x) = \left(\sum_{j=1}^{n} w_{jk}x_j + b_k \right) \qquad (1)$$

Where f (w,x,b)) is the activation function.

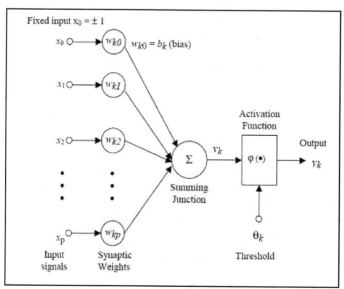

Fig. 3. Nonlinear model of a neuron

In general , there are four basic types of activation functions:

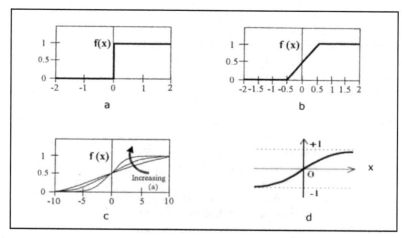

Fig. 4. Activation Functions

The management of neurons into layers and the connection patterns within and between layers is called the net architecture. The manner in which the neurons of a neural network are structured is intimately linked with the learning algorithms used to train the network [11]. Fig (5) shows different closes of network architecture

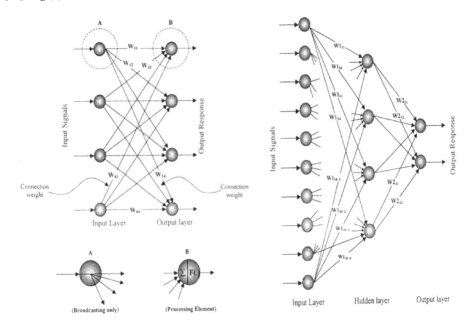

Fig. 5.a. Single-Layer Feedforward Networks b. Multilayer Feedforward Networks

2.2 Genetic algorithms
A genetic algorithm (GA) is a search heuristic that mimics the process of natural evolution. This heuristic is routinely used to generate useful solutions to optimization and search problems. Genetic algorithms belong to the larger class of evolutionary algorithms (EA), which generate solutions to optimization problems using techniques inspired by natural evolution, such as inheritance, mutation, selection, and crossover.In a genetic algorithm, a population of strings (called chromosomes or the genotype of the genome), which encode candidate solutions (called individuals, creatures, or phenotypes) to an optimization problem, evolves toward better solutions. Traditionally, solutions are represented in binary as strings of 0s and 1s, but other encodings are also possible. The evolution usually starts from a population of randomly generated individuals and happens in generations. In each generation, the fitness of every individual in the population is evaluated, multiple individuals are stochastically selected from the current population (based on their fitness), and modified (recombined and possibly randomly mutated) to form a new population. The new population is then used in the next iteration of the algorithm. Commonly, the algorithm terminates when either a maximum number of generations has been produced, or a satisfactory fitness level has been reached for the population. If the algorithm has terminated due to a maximum number of generations, a satisfactory solution may or may not have been reached.

Genetic algorithms find application in bioinformatics, phylogenetics, computational science, engineering, economics, chemistry, manufacturing, mathematics, physics and other fields. A typical genetic algorithm requires:

- a genetic representation of the solution domain,
- a fitness function to evaluate the solution domain.

A standard representation of the solution is as an array of bits. Arrays of other types and structures can be used in essentially the same way. The main property that makes these genetic representations convenient is that their parts are easily aligned due to their fixed size, which facilitates simple crossover operations. Variable length representations may also be used, but crossover implementation is more complex in this case. Tree-like representations are explored in genetic programming and graph-form representations are explored in evolutionary programming.[12]

The fitness function is defined over the genetic representation and measures the quality of the represented solution. The fitness function is always problem dependent. For instance, in the knapsack problem one wants to maximize the total value of objects that can be put in a knapsack of some fixed capacity. A representation of a solution might be an array of bits, where each bit represents a different object, and the value of the bit (0 or 1) represents whether or not the object is in the knapsack. Not every such representation is valid, as the size of objects may exceed the capacity of the knapsack. The fitness of the solution is the sum of values of all objects in the knapsack if the representation is valid, or 0 otherwise. In some problems, it is hard or even impossible to define the fitness expression; in these cases, interactive genetic algorithms are used.

Once we have the genetic representation and the fitness function defined, GA proceeds to initialize a population of solutions randomly, then improve it through repetitive application of mutation, crossover, inversion and selection operators as shown in fig 6.

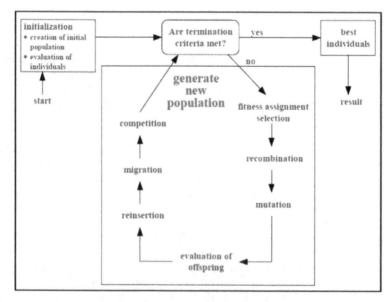

Fig. 6. Structure of an extended multi-population evolutionary algorithm

2.3 Fuzzy logic

Fuzzy logic [13] deals with fuzzy sets and logical connectives for modeling the human-like reasoning problems of the real world. A fuzzy set, unlike conventional sets, includes all elements of the universal set of the domain but with varying membership values in the interval [0,1]. It may be noted that a conventional set contains its members with a value of membership equal to one and disregards other elements of the universal set, for they have zero membership.

Fuzzy Sets and Crisp sets: The very basic notion of fuzzy systems is a fuzzy (sub)set. In classical mathematics we are familiar with what we call crisp sets. For example, the possible interferometric coherence g values are the set X of all real numbers between 0 and 1. From this set X a subset A can be defined, (e.g. all values $0 \leq g \geq 0.2$). The characteristic function of A, (i.e. this function assigns a number 1 or 0 to each element in X, depending on whether the element is in the subset A or not) is shown in fig7.[14]

The elements which have been assigned the number 1 can be interpreted as the elements that are in the set A and the elements which have assigned the number 0 as the elements that are not in the set A.

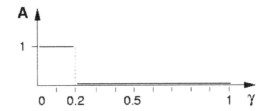

Fig. 7. Characteristic Function of a Crisp Set

This concept is sufficient for many areas of applications, but it can easily be seen, that it lacks in flexibility for some applications like classification of remotely sensed data analysis. For example it is well known that water shows low interferometric coherence g in SAR images. Since g starts at 0, the lower range of this set ought to be clear. The upper range, on the other hand, is rather hard to define. As a first attempt, we set the upper range to 0.2. Therefore we get B as a crisp interval B=[0,0.2]. But this means that a g value of 0.20 is low but a g value of 0.21 not. Obviously, this is a structural problem, for if we moved the upper boundary of the range from g =0.20 to an arbitrary point we can pose the same question. A more natural way to construct the set B would be to relax the strict separation between low and not low. This can be done by allowing not only the crisp decision Yes/No, but more flexible rules like " fairly low". A fuzzy set allows us to define such a notion. The aim is to use fuzzy sets in order to make computers more 'intelligent', therefore, the idea above has to be coded more formally. In the example, all the elements were coded with 0 or 1. A straight way to generalize this concept, is to allow more values between 0 and 1. In fact, infinitely many alternatives can be allowed between the boundaries 0 and 1, namely the unit interval I = [0, 1].

The interpretation of the numbers, now assigned to all elements is much more difficult. Of course, again the number 1 assigned to an element means, that the element is in the set B and 0 means that the element is definitely not in the set B. All other values mean a gradual membership to the set B.

This is shown in Fig. 8. The membership function is a graphical representation of the magnitude of participation of each input. It associates a weighting with each of the inputs that are processed, define functional overlap between inputs, and ultimately determines an output response. The rules use the input membership values as weighting factors to determine their influence on the fuzzy output sets of the final output conclusion.

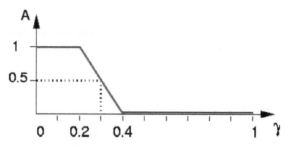

Fig. 8. Characteristic Function of a Fuzzy Set

Operations on fuzzy sets: We can introduce basic operations on fuzzy sets. Similar to the operations on crisp sets we also want to intersect, unify and negate fuzzy sets. In his very first paper about fuzzy sets [14], L. A. Zadeh suggested the minimum operator for the intersection and the maximum operator for the union of two fuzzy sets. It can be shown that these operators coincide with the crisp unification, and intersection if we only consider the membership degrees 0 and 1. For example, if A is a fuzzy interval between 5 and 8 and B be a fuzzy number about 4 as shown in the fig. 9.

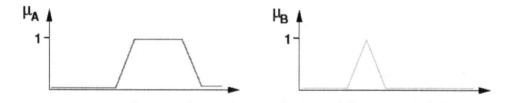

Fig. 9. Example fuzzy sets

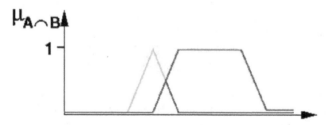

Fig. 10. Example: Fuzzy AND

In this case, the fuzzy set between 5 and 8 AND about 4 is set between 5 and 8 OR about 4 is shown in fig 11, and the the NEGATION of the fuzzy set A is shown in fig 12.

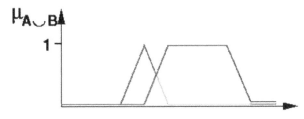

Fig. 11. Example: Fuzzy OR

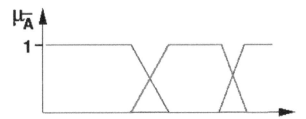

Fig. 12. Example: Fuzzy NEGATION

Fuzzy Classification: Fuzzy classifiers are one application of fuzzy theory. Expert knowledge is used and can be expressed in a very natural way using linguistic variables , which are described by fuzzy sets Now the expert knowledge for this variables can be formulated as a rules like
IF feature A low AND feature B medium AND feature C medium AND feature D medium THEN Class = class4
The rules can be combined in a table calls rule base [14]

R#	Feature A	Feature B	Feature C	Feature D	Class
1:	Low	Medium	Medium	Medium	Class 1
2:	Medium	high	Medium	Medium	Class 2
3:	Low	Medium	Medium	Medium	Class 3
4:	low	Medium	Medium	Medium	Class 1
5:	Medium	Medium	Medium	Medium	Class 4
...:	...	...	...	...	...
N:	Low	High	Medium	Low	Unknown

Linguistic rules describing the control system consist of two parts; an antecedent block (between the IF and THEN) and a consequent block (following THEN). Depending on the system, it may not be necessary to evaluate every possible input combination, since some may rarely or never occur.[14].

By making this type of evaluation, usually done by an experienced operator, fewer rules can be evaluated, thus simplifying the processing logic and perhaps even improving the fuzzy logic system performance. The inputs are combined logically using the AND operator to produce output response values for all expected inputs. The active conclusions are then combined into a logical sum for each membership function. A firing strength for each output membership function is computed. All that remains is to combine these logical sums in a defuzzification process to produce the crisp output. e.g for a for the rule consequents for each class a so-called singleton or a min–max interference can be derived which is the characteristic function of the respective set . e.g. For the input pair of H = 0:35 and _ = 30 the scheme below (see Fig 14.) would apply.

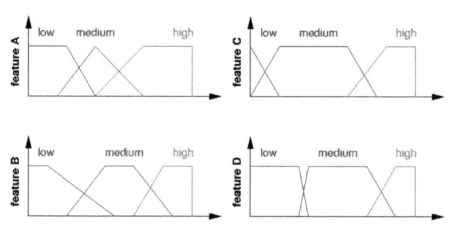

Fig. 13. Example: Linguistic Variables

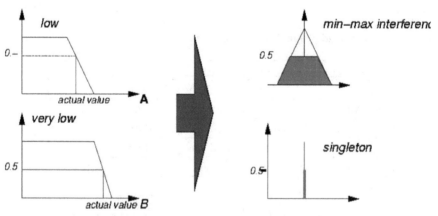

Fig. 14. Interference for rule IF H very low AND a low THEN Class = class 1

The fuzzy outputs for all rules are finally aggregated to one fuzzy set. To obtain a crisp decision from this fuzzy output, we have to defuzzify the fuzzy set, or the set of singletons. Therefore, we have to choose one representative value as the final output. There are several heuristic methods (defuzzification methods), one of them is e.g. to take the center of gravity of the fuzzy set as shown in fig 15., which is widely used for fuzzy sets. For the discrete case with singletons usually the maximum-method is used where the point with the maximum singleton is chosen.

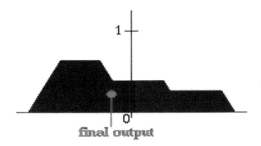

Fig. 15. Defuzzification using the center of gravity approach

3. Applications of AI techniques

Almost every branch of science and engineering currently shares the tools and techniques available in the domain of AI. However, we mention here a few typical applications, [15-20].
Expert Systems: An expert system consists of a knowledge base, database and an inference engine for interpreting the database using the knowledge supplied in the knowledge base.
Image Understanding and Computer Vision: A digital image can be regarded as a two-dimensional array of pixels containing gray levels corresponding to the intensity of the reflected illumination received by a video camera .
Navigational Planning for Mobile Robots: Mobile robots, sometimes called automated guided vehicles (AGV), are a challenging area of research where AI finds extensive applications. The navigational planning problem persists in both static and dynamic environments.
Speech Understanding: the main problem is to separate the syllables of a spoken word and determine features like amplitude, and fundamental and harmonic frequencies of each syllable. The words then could be identified from the Extracted features by pattern classification techniques.
Scheduling: In a scheduling problem, one has to plan the time schedule of a set of events to improve the time efficiency of the solution.
Intelligent Control: In process control, the controller is designed from the known models of the process and the required control objective. When the dynamics of the plant is not completely known, the existing techniques for controller design no longer remain valid. Rule-based control is appropriate in such situations.
System Modeling and Optimization:
Optimization methods have been applied over years to generate solutions that solely maximize performance. In order to assess the performance variance of a solution, a few near optimal solutions are selected and studied under assumed stochastic parametric variations via simulation. There are reports on the use AI guide or bias search strategies. A new evolutionary algorithm that is capable of generating robust optimal solutions for constrained robust design problems.

3.1 Using AI for medical applications

The implementation of human intelligence in scientific equipment has been the subject of scientific research for a long time and of the medical research in the last decades. In the 1950's computer simulation of biological neural network was first introduced. In 1943 McCullogh and Pitts stated the definition of the first artificial neuron. In parallel with the evolution of computer technology, modeling of increasingly complicated neural functions and activity of simple neural clusters was defined. Mathematical models that could be applied for practical applications were developed between 1982 and 1987 based on the works of Hopfield [21], Kohonen [22] and Rummelhart and McLelland [23]. The advantage of neural networks over conventional programming lies in their ability to solve problems that do not have an algorithmic solution or the available solution is too complex to be found. Neural networks are well suited to tackle problems that people are good at solving, such as prediction and pattern recognition. Neural networks have been applied within the medical domain for clinical diagnosis [24-26], image analysis and interpretation[27,28] signal analysis and interpretation [29] and drug development [30]..

Functional division of neural network applications in medicine; Papik et al, 1998) [31]:

1. Modelling: Simulating and modelling the functions of the brain and neurosensory organs.
2. Signal processing: Bioelecric signal filtering and evaluation.
3. System control and checking: Intelligent artificial machine control and checking based on responses of biological or technical systems given to any signals
4. Classification: Interpretation of physical and instrumental findings to achieve more accurate diagnosis.
5. Prediction: Neural network provide prognostic information based on retrospective parameter analysis.

Fuzzy logic [11] has been applied to dental and medical sciences n3(Sims-Williams et al, 1987) in order to construct systems that can infer precise recommendations for solving problems that have uncertain properties [32-36] .Brown et al. (1991) [37] applied fuzzy logic to solve orthodontic problems in an expert system, designed to provide advice for treatment planning of Class II division 1 malocclusions. They reported that their system produced more acceptable treatment plans than those used by general dental practitioners. Similarly, Tanaka et al. (1997) [36] applied fuzzy reasoning to their computer-assisted diagnostic system for ultrasonography for the purpose of providing a diagnostic aid for unskilled clinicians.(head gear)

4. Using AI for orthodontics

Many researchers intended to capture the outlines matching between pleasing smile and harmonically face. Usually the challenging face the orthodontist to figure out the orthodontic problems, there diagnosis and environment of origin keeping away distracting factors. The traditional regime for diagnosis include multiple steps for orthodontic problem identification , these steps generally categorized according to three sources (1) multiple questioning records including chief complaint, patient's dental and medical history; (2) clinical examination of the patient; and (3) assessment of diagnostic records, including dental casts, radiographs, and facial and intraoral images [38].

It is mandatory to contextualize data have been driven. All the data base collected gathered in an elaborate process to achieve the most appropriate treatment planning, treatment plan is the second challenge facing the orthodontist, the enormous variation in dental malocclusion gathered with different facial pattern and the presence of large number of available treatment modalities, all these leading the decision process in orthodontics to challenging area even to the experienced orthodontist. Often more than one treatment plan can successfully resolve an orthodontic problem, and as a consequences form these two interrelated orthodontic processes (diagnosis and treatment plan) the treatment can be customized , orthodontic books and articles are profound with researches discussing protocols for decision making process regarding orthodontic problem definition and treatment option. Thus our chapter attempt to bring the insight to the invention of the artificial intelligence as a system aid in the essential orthodontic steps namely; diagnosis, treatment plan and treatment optimization.

4.1 Diagnosis using expert system

Expert system (ES) is an important branch of the field of artificial intelligence (AI).. ES is a computer program system that processes knowledge and information, which is composed primarily of a knowledge base and an inference machine. ES simulates the decision making and working processes of experts and solves actual problems in the field of a single specialty[39]. Generally, in a medical or dental expert system, a set of knowledge base is derived from experienced clinicians and represents their knowledge, which can be used for clinical consultations [40,41].With this type of system, uncertainty is a major problem in decision making because non-evidence-based knowledge has to be represented mathematically. Poon et al [42] were the first to use a new approach to knowledge acquisition known as Ripple-Down Rules in Dentistry to develop an ES in clinical orthodontics. This system comprises a knowledge base of 680 rules. Investigators found that such an ES has potential as an interactive advisory tool and is applicable in clinical orthodontic situations.

Hammond et al [43] pointed out in a review that traditional rule-based expert systems had some limitations when applied to orthodontic diagnosis and treatment planning. These limitations may be avoided by using a case-based system, which is a particular type of ES that uses a stored data bank of previously treated cases to provide knowledge for use in solving new treatment problems. Hammond et al [44] also investigated the application of this method in the field of orthodontic diagnosis and treatment planning. A case base of 300 cases was entered into a case based ES shell. A test set of 30 consecutive cases then was used to test the diagnostic capacity of the system. The computer-generated treatment plan matched the actual treatment plan in 24 of the 30 cases. In another work by Lux et al [45] the growth of 43 orthodontically untreated children was analyzed by lateral cephalograms taken at the ages of 7 and 15. For the description of craniofacial skeletal changes, the concept of tensor analysis and related methods were applied. Through the use of an ANN, namely, self-organizing neural maps (SOM), resultant growth data were classified, and relationships of the various growth patterns were monitored. This type of network provided a frame of reference for classifying and analyzing previously unknown cases with respect to their growth pattern, Brickley et al [46] concluded that ANN expert systems may be trained with clinical data only and therefore can be used in cases where "rule-based" decision making is not possible. This is the case in many clinical situations. ANN therefore may become important decision-making tools within dentistry, we'll discuss one of these expert systems;

An expert orthodontic index:

A valid initial assessment enables health providers to determine treatment need and priority, an accurate final diagnostic assessment assists patients and orthodontists to conclude if a worthwhile improvement is achieved. Orthodontists have developed several occlusal indices during the past few decades to evaluate treatment need, complexity, and success. Among the developed indices, Peer Assessment Rating (PAR) is one of the most common ones that is used to evaluate the quality of treatment. Richmond et al [47] developed PAR in 1992 to create consistency and standardization in assessing orthodontic treatment outcome. It is a weighted summation of health traits that influence the malocclusion. It summarizes data about the misalignment in a single score that reflects deviation from the ideal occlusion. The treatment success can then be evaluated by comparison of the pre- and post-treatment PAR scores. In spite of its extensive use, PAR suffers from several limitations. In summary, PAR is constrained by its strict linear mathematical expression with fixed coefficients, while a non-linearity may enhance the subjective opinions of orthodontists more accurately. Different versions of PAR index have been developed in order to improve the weighting system by using traditional regression techniques, but they are still restricted by the non-adjustable linear coefficient. A fuzzy index was developed by Zarei A.et al in 2007[48] using neural network with fuzzy approach . Zarei et al in 2009 [49] improved the quality of fuzzy index using union rule configuration. Further, an intelligent system that represent orthodontists' visual perception in assessing patients was developed.

Panel of orthodontists with randomized patients' files, each of which contained their data prior to treatment, during treatment progress, and at the end of treatment. profiles of 560 cases of malocclusion was used by the panel of orthodontist . each profile includes clinician's assessment that based on cephalometric tracing interpretations, visual perception, and clinical appearance. The panel assessed the cases using a visual analog scale. A visual analog scale is one of the most common measurement scales used in health care research and has also been used in dental studies [50].

Modeling was used for the identification of the expert system using the input-output data. Sugeno models [51] are good candidates for situations when a desired action can not necessarily be described verbally by experts. Therefore, Sugeno models provide a good way to model clinicians' assessment when using numerical data. a set of input-output data to first identify the fuzzy system for this collection of data and then optimize this model by adjusting the parameters. Input to this fuzzy inference model includes five variables that orthodontists associate with assessment of treatment outcome, The input variables for this model include the following linear and angular cephalometric measurements; overjet, ANB angle, Lower Incisor to Mandibular Plane angle (LI-MnPl), SNB angle and Upper Incisor to Sella Nasion angle (UI-SN),while the output parameter is the arithmetic mean of the panel's assessments. Subtractive clustering to identify the rule base was performed, clustering of data forms the basis of many system modeling algorithms.

Neural networks were utilized to learn the characteristics of the data and selected the parameters of input and output membership functions to best reflect those characteristics. The parameters of membership functions are modified during the learning process to minimize the fitness function. The adjustments of these parameters are facilitated by a gradient vector, which provides a measure of how well the fuzzy inference system is modeling the data. Optimization of the parameters of the initial model with respect to training data by minimizing the sum of the squared difference between actual and desired outputs. Fig 16 depicts the performance of the model in predicting the assessment for training and testing patterns. It is evident from this figure that the model assessment is very close to the panel assessment for most of the patterns.

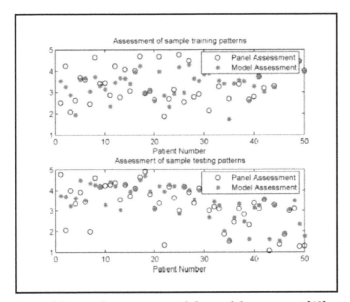

Fig. 16. Comparison of the panel assessment and the model assessment [49]

a Neuro-Fuzzy Assessment Index that is highly correlated with clinicians' opinion were successfully produced. neural network and fuzzy logic had been used for assessing orthodontic treatment outcome and developed a robust and realistic model that has a flexible interpretation of data. Applying Subtractive Clustering technique avoided the combinatorial explosion of rules in our model. hybridization of neural network and fuzzy logic improved the quality of the orthodontic index.[52].

Cephalometrics Analysis

Cephalometric analysis is a useful diagnostic tool to determine facial type and prediction of growth pattern, enabling clinician to determine facial disharmonies in order to centralize therapeutic measures during treatment and modify facial growth.

According to Graber and Vanarsdall [38], the commonly used radiographic views are:

Lateral or profile cephalograms: used to study anteroposterior and vertical relationships.

Frontal or postero-anterior celphalograms: used to evaluate the transversal and vertical relationships in the frontal plane. Submentovertex or basal cephalograms: used to the balance in transversal plane.

Two approaches may be used to perform a cephalometric analysis: a manual approach, and a computer- aided approach. The manual approach is the oldest and most widely used. It consists of placing a sheet of acetate over the cephalometric radiograph, tracing salient features, identifying landmarks, and measuring distances and angles between landmark locations. The other approach is computer-aided. Computerized cephalometric analysis uses manual identification of landmarks, based either on an overlay tracing of the radiograph to identify anatomical or constructed points followed by the transfer of the tracing to a digitizer linked to a computer, or a direct digitization of the lateral skull radiograph using a digitizer linked to a computer, and then locating landmarks on the monitor.[42-44].

Afterwards, the computer software completes the cephalometric analysis by automatically measuring distances and angles. The evolution from full manual cephalometrics to computer assisted-cephalometric analysis is aimed at improving the diagnostic ability of cephalometric analysis through errors reduction and time saving. Computerized or computer-aided, cephalometric analysis eliminates the mechanical errors when drawing lines between landmarks as well as those made when measuring with a protractor. However, the inconsistency in landmark identification is still an important source of random errors both in computer-aided digital cephalometry and in manual cephalometric analysis.[45-47] taking into account the imprecise, inconsistent, and paracomplete data inherent to the analytical process. There have been efforts to automate cephalometric analysis with the aim of reducing the time required to obtain an analysis, improving the accuracy of landmark identification and reducing the errors due to clinicians' subjectivity.

In an automated cephalometric analysis a scanned or digital cephalometric radiograph is stored in the computer and loaded by the software. The software then automatically locates the landmarks and performs the measurements for cephalometric analysis. The challenging problem in an automated cephalometric analysis is landmark detection, given that the calculations have already been automated with success. The first attempt at automated landmarking of cephalograms was made by Cohen in 1984,[53] ,followed by more studies on this topic. Automatic identification of landmarks has been undertaken in different ways that involve computer vision and artificial intelligence techniques.

The automated approaches can be classified into four broad categories, based on the techniques, Leonardia R et al[54] mentioned these categories with techniques examples for each approach recorded by different authors:

1.   Image filtering plus knowledge-based landmark search; [55-58]
2.   model- based approaches [59-64]
3.   soft-computing approaches [65-68]
4.   hybrid approaches. [69-73]

the relative advantages and disadvantages of these technical approaches used in the automated identification of cephalometric landmarks; Image filtering plus knowledge-based landmark search are list in table 1.

The informational importance of the cephalometric analysis was accompanied by many unnegligible sites of imprecision, this significant degrees of vagueness, and even inconsistency, was also making clinical application of the cephalometric data interpretation and driven information of less effective values than expected by the clinicians. to interpret how cephalometric variables behave in a complete contextualized scenario. Many trials was made to extract the ability of artificial intelligent techniques as favorable interpretational tool for the usual inconsistency of biological information. As a matter of fact artificial intelligence (AI) theories or techniques have few and recent applications in craniofacial biology, specifically in clinical application of cephalometrics, the multiple discussed studies was successfully produced at the level of researches taking in to account that the systems described in the literature are not accurate enough to allow their use for clinical purposes as errors in landmark detection were greater than those expected with manual tracing, therefore; most of these methods have not been adopted in clinical practice [53]. The inconsistency of the informational driven cephalometric data gave the authors an additional challenging interface to overcome both cephalometric and modeling techniques inconsistencies, and yields sequential attempts of automated cephalometric analysis; we'll discuss some of these attempts in details hoping the enrichment of reader information of artificial intelligent approach for this diagnostic tool;

Techniques	Advantages	Disadvantages
Image filtering plus knowledge-based landmark search	Easy to implement Image filtering techniques are well studied and a large number are available By encoding proper anatomical knowledge better accuracy	Can fail to capture morphological variability in the radiographs Filtering results are highly dependent on image quality and intensity level Sensitive to noise in the image. Not all landmarks lie on edge and, moreover, the edges or curve are often unclear.
Model-based approach	Is invariant to scale, rotation, and translation (the structure can be located even if it is smaller or bigger than given model). Accommodates shape variability	Needs models that must be created by averaging the variations in shape of each anatomical structure on given set of radiographs. Model deformation must be constrained and is not always precise Cannot be applied to partially hidden regions Sensitive to noise in image.
Soft-computing or learning approach	Accommodates shape variability. Tolerant to noise. Techniques are well studies. Large selection of software tools available.	Results depend on the training set. Difficult to interpret some results. A number of network parameters, such as topology and number of neuron must be determined empirically.

Table 1. Technical approaches used to automatically identify cephalometric landmarks and their advantages and disadvantages [54].

Abe [74] and Mario et al [75]mentioned important limitations that conventional cephalometric holds, mostly due to the fact that the cephalometric variables are not assessed under a contextualized scope and carry on important variation when compared to samples norms. Because of that, its clinical application is subjective. Also discordance between orthodontists about diagnosis and treatments it is not uncommon, due to the inevitable uncertainties involved in the cephalometrics variables, and both suggest that this is a perfect scenario to evaluate the paraconsistent neural network capacity to perform with uncertainties, and inconsistencies in a practical problem.

Abe [74] develops an expert system in his work to support orthodontic diagnosis, the system based on the paraconsistent approach. Paraconsistent artificial neural network (PANN) was introduced in the Bulletin of Symbolic Logic [74], In the structure proposed the inferences that were based upon the degrees of evidence (favorable and unfavorable) of abnormality for cephalometrics variables, which may have infinite values between "0" and "1", the suggested PANN refined in Abe [74] work to produce an expert system to support orthodontic diagnosis, which may have infinite values between "0" and "1". Therefore, the system may be refined with more or less outputs, depending upon the need. Such flexibility allows that the system can be modeled in different ways, allowing a finer adjusting. The system requires measurements taken from the head lateral radiography of the patient that will be assessed. The precision of the system increase as much as data is added.

Another work was made by Mario et al [75] to overcome these interpretational shortcomings, once again suggesting the contribution of Mathematics to Biology, better translating natural phenomena. Moreover, single correlations are insufficient for the assessment of facial patterns as many variables must be simultaneously considered in order to establish patterns. And once again the paraconsistent logic suggested as a model for detection and treatment of contradictions, enriching the use of soft mathematics tools in biology. research intends to test such model, it is reasonable to expect that the proposed model can well detect inconsistencies and better interpret craniofacial morphology [75], the cephalometric diagnostic model used logical states which represented in figure 7.

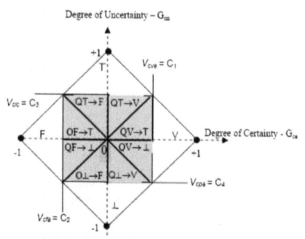

Fig. 17. Logical states: extreme and nonextreme states [75]

PANN

PANN was introduced in the *Bulletin of Symbolic Logic* (10). Its basis leans on paraconsistent annotated evidential logic Eτ(10). Let us present it briefly. The atomic formulas of the logic Et are of the type

$p(\mu, \lambda)$, where $p(\mu, \lambda)$, $\in[0, 1]^2$ and [0, 1] is the real unitary nterval (p denotes a propositional variable).The $p(\mu, \lambda)$, can be intuitively read: "It is assumed that p's favorable i.evidence is μ and contrary evidence is λ. Thus,

- $p(1.0, 0.0)$ can be read as a true proposition;
- $p(0.0, 1.0)$ can be read as a false proposition;
- $p(1.0, 1.0)$ can be read as an inconsistent proposition;
- $p(0.0, 0.0)$ can be read as a paracomplete (unknown) proposition;
- $p(0.5, 0.5)$ can be read as an indefinite proposition.

In the PANN, the main aim is to know how to determine the certainty degree concerning a proposition, if it is False or True. Therefore, the model took the certainty degree Gce into account. The uncertainty degree Gun indicates the "measure" of the inconsistency or paracompleteness [78]. If the certainty degree is low or the uncertainty degree is high, it generates an indefinition; the basic scheme is shown in Fig. 18.

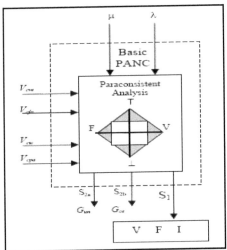

Fig. 18. The basic steps of a paraconsistent artificial neural cell

The model suggested by Mario et al [75] utilize selected set of cephalometric variables based on expertise (Figs. 9 a and b). These cephalometric variables are usually collected by experts [79] through characteristic points in a cephalometric X-ray.

The selected cephalometric variables feed the PANN in the following three units: Unit I, considering the anteroposterior discrepancy; Unit II, considering vertical discrepancy; and Unit III, taking into account dental discrepancy (see Fig. 20).

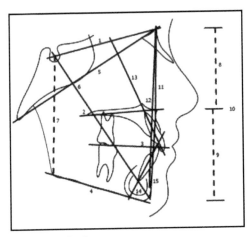

Fig. 19. a Cephalometric Variables [73]

(1. Basion 2. Sella 3. Nasion 4. Posterior Nasal Spine 5. Anterior Nasal Spine 6. Inter-Molars 7. Inter-Incisors 8. Gonion 9. Menton 10. Gnathion 11. A Point 12. B Point 13. Pogonion 14. Incisal Edge - Upper Incisor 15. Apex - Upper Incisor 16. Incisal Edge - Lower Incisor 17. Apex - Lower Incisor)

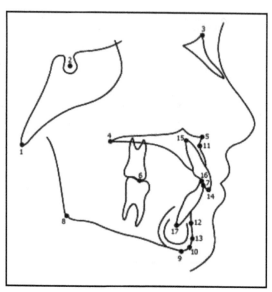

Fig. 19. b Proposed Cephalometric Analysis [73]

1. Anterior Cranial Base 2. Palatal Plane (PP) 3. Oclusal Plane (OP) 4. Mandibular Plane (MP) 5. Cranial Base 6. Y Axis 7. Posterior Facial Height 8. Anterior Facial Height - Median Third 9. Anterior Facial Height - Lower Third 10. Anterior Facial Height 11. SNA 12. SNB 13. Long Axis - Upper Incisor 14. Long Axis - Lower Incisor 15. A Point - Pogonion Line Wits: distance between the projections of the A and B Points on the occlusal plane.

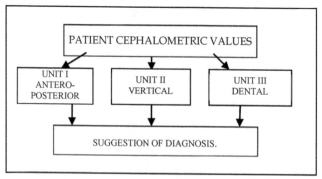

Fig. 20. Functional macroview of the paraconsistent artificial neural network architecture used by Mario et al [75]

Each unit has the specific following components, as shown in Fig 21:

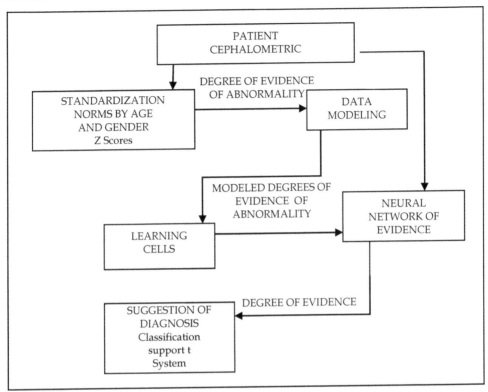

Fig. 21. Functional microview of the structure of each unit represented in Fig. 20 [75]

Tanikawa C etal [80] studied the reliability of a system that performs automatic recognition of anatomic landmarks and their surrounding anatomic structures in which the landmarks are located on lateral cephalograms using landmark-dependent criteria unique to each respective landmark. Recently, a system that recognizes general grayscale images using an automated psychologic brain model [81] has been developed.ie, a hardware-friendly algorithm to accomplish real-time recognition by recalling a set of modeled data that is mathematically described using a finite number of traits and previously stored in the system. This system employs a new technique called the projected principal edge distribution (PPED) as a means for extracting features from an image, and it has been confirmed that the system demonstrates robust performance in recognizing images, including cephalograms [82-84]. Although experiments have suggested the efficacy of the system in recognizing images, it remains uncertain whether such a system will detect conventionally used landmarks with high precision. On the other hand, as mentioned before, that topographic variations exist in humans' subjective judgments of cephalometric landmarks, and the shapes and size of the variances are unique to each landmark [85]. Mathematical formulation of these landmark-dependent variations in measurement would be help researchers to evaluate objectively the reliability of the automatic cephalogram recognition system.

Tanikawa C et al [80] system incorporates two major tasks: the "knowledge-generation" (system learning) phase and the "recognition" phase. In the knowledge generation phase, image data extracted from learning asamples are converted into PPED vectors consisting of 64 variables that feature contours of the anatomic structures [81,82,83] .From these vectors, template vectors, i.e., the principal information for identifying the landmarks, are generated using a generalized Lloyd algorithm [86] for each landmark, which are stored in the system as the system's knowledge. During the recognition phase, the system is designed to perform pixel- by-pixel film scanning with template-matching operations between PPED vectors that are generated from an input film and template vectors stored on the system. The system recognizes the most matched position as a landmark position. schematic representation can be seen in fig 22.

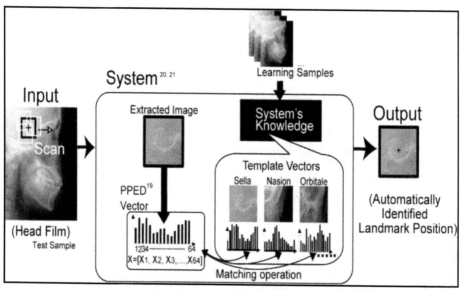

Fig. 22. Schematic representation for automatic recognition of anatomic landmarks [80]

To evaluate the system's performance reliability, scattergrams that designated errors for manual landmark identification when 10 orthodontists identified a landmark on 10 cephalograms were obtained according to the method reported by Baumrind and Frantz [85]. Confidence ellipses with a confidence limit of α were developed for each landmark from the scattergram, the system was evaluated using confidence ellipses with α =.01 In short, when a system-identified point was located within a confidence limit of α = .01, the landmark identification was judged to be successful.

To evaluate the accuracy of the landmark identification provided by the systems and if system's definition of a landmark position is clinically acceptable, it has been a critical issue in testing the performance reliability of such systems. Three major methods for such an evaluation have been employed so far. In the first method, an individual orthodontist makes a visual judgment as to whether or not the system's recommendation is acceptable [87] The second approach involves describing mean recognition errors, i.e., the mean distance between the point provided by an orthodontist(s) and the point determined by the system [88,89]. The third method is to examine whether the system-identified landmark is located in a circle with a 2-mm radius [88-93], see fig13.

The fiducial zones established by the panel of experienced orthodontists are considered valid for evaluation of the ability of the automatic recognition system to recognize anatomic features. With the incorporation of the rational assessment criteria provided by confidence ellipses, the proposed system was confirmed to be reliable. The system successfully recognized anatomic features surrounding all the landmarks. The mean success rate for identifying the landmark positions was 88% with a range of 77% to 100%.

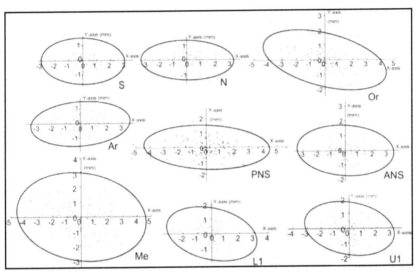

Fig. 23. Confidence ellipses obtained for cephalometric landmarks. Black points indicate coordinate values of landmarks identified by 10 orthodontists on 10 cephalograms. The black lines designate confidence ellipses with α=01. Origin indicates the best estimate; x-axis, the line that passes through the origin and is parallel to the line S-N; and y-axis, the line that is perpendicular to the x-axis through the origin. [80].

In 2011 Banumathi A et al suggested [94] Another diagnostic model, Artificial intelligence role in dentofacial deformities diagnosis was discussed. The dentist must be familiar with morphological and functional maturity also oral surgeon and the orthodontist should be able to relate this knowledge to specific clinical problems such as skeletal mealocclusion and craniofacial anomalies. This understanding should influence the selection, planning and timing of treatment for patients who require orthognathic surgery. And the decision forming through the available choices, whether accepting the underlying deformity and taking the camouflage treatment as a choice or maybe surgical correction is the sole solution could be offered, of course   full awareness of patient psychological aspects, underlying skeletal and\or dental malrelations and specific age, all should be taken into account. Cephalometric analysis was of important priority in deciding the acceptance and selection of appropriate orhognathic surgery for the underlying case. the diagnostic model was proposed by Edge sharpening of various bones in the lateral view of the face in cephalometric image referred to preprocessing, this is achieved through a histogram equalization process. From the literature, histogram equalization is enough to improve the contrast of the cephalometric image [95]. The edge features are then extracted from the enhanced cephalometric image and they are classified as landmark and non landmark points using Support vector machine technique. Finally, angles between various landmark points are calculated to find out the deformities in the dento-facial growth. Banumathi A. et al [94] used in this study the Projected Principal Edge Distribution (PPED) vectors as a system for medical image recognition, and was used also in image recognition system dicussed above described by Tanikawa C et al [80], as this techniques proved to provide better results.

4.2 Planning of treatment using AI

Enormous amount of variant subjects lies in the etiological list of orthodontic problems, we'll try at this section to show the artificial intelligent task in the planning of appropriate therapeutic goals can be achieved within certain boundaries for each problem, these boundaries considers the available problematic outcomes and its related factor as the backbone of system modeling and comparing these treatment plan with authors subjective opinions to simulate the treatment plan created by human brain.

Cranifacial Growth modification

Planning of treatment in the field of orthodontics and maxillo-facial surgery is largely dependent on the classification of individual growth of a patient. Work by Lux CJ et al[45] suggested the use of an artificial neural network, namely self-organizing neural maps, the growth of 43 orthodontically untreated children was analyzed by means of lateral cephalograms taken at the ages of 7 and 15. For the description of craniofacial skeletal changes, the concept of tensor analysis and related methods have been applied. Thus the geometric and analytical limitations of conventional cephalometric methods have been avoided, the resultant growth data were classified and the relationships of the various growth patterns were monitored by using an artificial neural network. As a result of self-organization, the 43 children were topologically ordered on the emerging map according to their craniofacial size and shape changes during growth. As a new patient can be allocated on the map, this type of network provides a frame of reference for classifying and analysing previously unknown cases according to their growth pattern. The morphometric methods applied as well as the subsequent visualization of the growth data by means of neural networks can be employed for the analysis and classification of growth-related skeletal changes in general.

Impacted canine

An impacted canine requires a complex therapeutic management, The therapeutic approach to impacted canines is interdisciplinary, with many factors accounting for the final orthodontic and periodontal outcomes. Pretreatment radiographic features of impacted canines—α-angle, d-distance, and sector of impaction according to Ericson and Kurol[96,97]have been shown to be predictive factors for the durations of orthodontic traction and comprehensive orthodontic treatment to reposition the impacted tooth. The more severely displaced the canine with regard to the adjacent maxillary incisors, the longer the orthodontic treatment[98], most investigations evaluated the relationships between factors accounting for treatment outcomes of impacted canines with descriptive statistics or linear regression on a priori identified variables; more recent studies used multilevel statistics to study associations among factors without determining causal relationships [99,100]. The multiple factors affecting the ultimate treatment approaches and duration should be included in the overall AI model. In 2010 Nieri M et al [101] used Bayesian networks (BN) to comprehensive surgical-orthodontic treatment of maxillary impacted canines to evaluate the relative role and the possible causal relationships among various factors affecting the clinical approach to this condition. BN adopt an intermediate approach between statistics and artificial intelligence. An automatic structural learning algorithm of the BN was used as an explorative statistical technique for detecting possible causal relationships among these variables:

demographic variables (sex and age);

topographic variables (clinical and radiographic): site (buccal or palatal), side (left or right), unilateral or bilateral (patient), a-angle, d-distance, s-sector; treatment technique (tunnel); duration of traction, duration of treatment; periodontal variables ; Width of keratinized tissue (KT), from the gingival margin to the mucogingival junction; and Probing depth (PD) measurements. These were evaluated for the treated teeth through the therapeutic course.

In the BN analysis. the metric variables were transformed into binary variables by using the median values as a threshold as shown in fig 24.

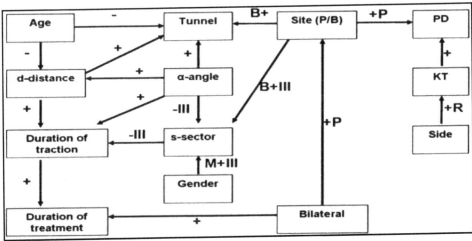

Fig. 24. The graph generated by the structural learning algorithm .P, Palatal; B, buccal; PD, probing depth; KT, keratinized tissue; R, right side; III, sector 3;M, male;1, the variable at the base of the arrow positively influences the variable at the arrowhead,the variable at the base of the arrow negatively influences the variable at the arrowhead, from Nieri M et al [101]

The BN approach confirmed the results of previous investigations on the same population in which the final periodontal outcomes after the surgical-orthodontic repositioning of maxillary impacted canines were unrelated to pretreatment diagnostic variables on the panoramic radiographs [100,102].The application of BN to diagnostic and therapeutic aspects of comprehensive surgical-orthodontic treatment of maxillary impacted canines identified several possible causal relationships among factors affecting the final outcomes of therapy.

Extraction demands in orthodontics

Early in the 20th century the maintaining of intact dentition became an important goal of orthodontic treatment. Angle and his followers strongly opposed extraction for orthodontic purposes. With the emphasis on dental occlusion that followed, however, less attention came to be paid to facial proportions and esthetics at that time. Small jaw size relative to the size of the teeth is an important factor in planning orthodontic therapy, as it implies that a significant percentage of patients will continue to require extractions to provide space for

aligning the remaining teeth. for over 100 years it has been a key question in planning orthodontic treatment. In orthodontics, there are two major reasons to extract teeth [103]:
1.   to provide space to align the remaining teeth in the presence of severe crowding, and
2.   to allow teeth to be moved (usually, incisors to be retracted) so protrusion can be reduced or so skeletal Class II or Class III problems can be camouflaged.
The alternative to extraction in treating dental crowding is to expand the arches; the alternative for skeletal problems is to correct the jaw relationship, by modifying growth or surgery. the majority of patients were treated with extractions to provide enough space for the other teeth. At present there again is great enthusiasm for expanding dental arches, on the theory that soft tissue adaptation will allow the expansion to be maintained, therefore; orthodontic treatments for malocclusion can be classified as extraction treatments and nonextraction treatments. The decision of extraction or not might be challenging and aimed to correct the malocclusion and enhancement of dental and facial appearance.

The decision to extract requires a multiple-factor analysis, which often includes the clinical experiences of the orthodontist. Currently, many multiple-factor analysis methods are available for use. Among these, the most frequently used is the statistical process known as fuzzy grouping analysis. Fuzzy grouping analysis regroups multiple factors based on their closeness in affecting the extraction decision. Classification by this algorithm is applicable to many patients. Xie X et al [39] study construct a decision-making expert system (ES) for orthodontic treatment by using a new approach. The ANN model was constructed to predict whether malocclusion patients between 11 and 15 years old required orthodontic extraction treatment. ANN model had 23 neurons in the input layer and 1 neuron in the output layer; this corresponded to the use of extraction or nonextraction treatments.

The model was implemented using the FORTRAN programming language, which is based on the principle of artificial neural networks. This Back Propagation (BP) ANN employs the error backward propagation learning algorithm. The basic principle of the BP algorithm is the propagation of errors from the output layer backward to the input layer by each layer that "shares" the error with neurons of each layer. Thus the reference errors of each layer of neuron are obtained for use in adjusting the corresponding connection weights, to make the error function diminish as far as possible. To enhance the performance of BP networks, a suitable learning parameter η and momentum parameter ε should be chosen properly. 25indices were selected for screening of subjects. Two of these were nonquantification indices, which included the situation of heredity and protruded anterior teeth uncovered by incompetent lips. Among the quantifiable indices, 5 were derived from cast measurement, 13 from hard tissue cephalometrics, and 5 from soft tissue cephalometrics.

Contributions of the 23 input layer indices to the output layer index were analyzed through the method of neural network data processing. The connection strengths of each neuron in the input layer with each neuron in the hidden layer were used to represent the values of contribution from every input index. The values of a new index F (i) were calculated respectively to represent the contributions. These new indices were ordered by their magnitude, with the largest on top. The new index described the contributions from every input index to the result, as is shown in Table 2. After the data were preprocessed, all input indices were valued at between 0 and 1. the output index was extraction or nonextraction, quantification was processed as 0.99 for "yes" and 0.01 for "no."

Data from the 180 patients-in-training set were used to train the ANN model described above. Data from 20 patients were used to test the accuracy of the ANN model. When η was chosen as 0.9 and ε as 0.7, and the number of neurons in the hidden layer was 13, the model had a nice learning effect. The 20 test samples proved successful in evaluating factors that affect the decision-making process. The rate of accuracy was 100%, which demonstrated that the constructed ANN could make correct decisions regarding the data of the trained 180 samples. Then, the data of 20 testing set samples that had not been trained were tested, and it demonstrated that the rate of accuracy was 80%. As for the marginal cases.

Input index	F(i)	order
Anterior teeth uncovered by incompetent lips	14042.44	1
IMPA (LI-MP)	11833.00	2
Overjet	6693.52	3
Crowding in the upper dental arch, mm	6135.12	4
Space for correction Sppe's curve, mm	5948.78	5
ANB	5891.38	6
Overbite	5689.83	7
LI-NB	5640.86	8
LL-E plane, mm	4697.43	9
Soft tissue convexity (Ns-Sn-Pos)	4033.89	10
Interincisal angle (UI-LI)	4000.84	11
UI-NA, mm	3967.02	12
Z angle	2872.43	13
Wits, mm	2664.37	14
NLA (Cm-Sn-UL)	2620.67	15
UI-SN	2447.43	16
UL-E plane, mm	2250.07	17
UI-NA	2199.48	18
Heredity	2190.95	19
Crowding in the lower dental arch, mm	2173.83	20
FMIA (L1-FH)	1966.10	21
L1-NB, mm	1520.10	22
FMA (FH-MP)	410.39	23

Table 2. Analysis of Contributions of Every Input Index used inXie X et al [39] expert system

Using AI in selecting the appropriate treatment modalities

a computer-assisted inference model for selecting appropriate types of headgear appliance for orthodontic patients and act as a decision-making aid for inexperienced clinicians was developed by Akgam M.O and Takada K [104] Headgear is mainly used in orthodontic practice to deliver extra-oral forces to the upper dental arch for anchorage purposes, distalizing teeth and/or inhibiting forward maxillary growth. It has three main types, i.e. low, medium, and high-pull describing the direction of force applied to the upper molar teeth in the sagittal plane[105]. The choice of the precise type of headgear may not be difficult when considering its application in 'typical' cases, such as those exhibiting a Class II malocclusion with a deep overbite, large over jet, and a low mandibular plane angle. A problem may arise, however, particularly for orthodontists who have less clinical experience, with 'borderline' or 'marginal' subjects, such as those having a deep overbite, a moderate to severe over jet, and a high mandibular plane angle. This is because decision making in choosing an appropriate headgear type cannot be dealt with in a discrete, but rather a continuous manner, i.e. *fuzzy logic.* the study incorporates three variables, namely, overjet, overbite, and mandibular plane angle, were used as input variables to the system. The mandibular plane angle was defined as the angle formed by the SN and mandibular planes. These variables were obtained from the lateral cephalograms.

For each input variable, three fuzzy sets for the low, medium, and high-pull types of headgear were defined on the basis of the authors' subjective judgment, which included their clinical experience and knowledge of the normative means and standard deviations for each variable. For each fuzzy set, the *fuzzy trapezoid function* was employed to construct membership functions. The fuzzy sets for each variable were determined with an assumption that the remaining two variables took normative values. For ease of understanding and simplicity, a graphic interpretation of the element and membership grade pairs which were created for the low, medium and high-pull types using each input variable is provided in Figures 25,26,27,Geometric mean aggregation was used for the inference, Geometric mean aggregation

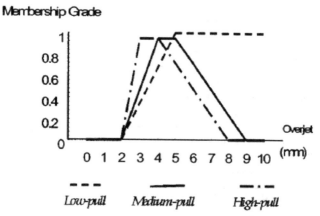

Fig. 25. Plot of membership functions for the input of overjet for each of three sets, i.e. the low-, medium-, and high-pull types of headgear.

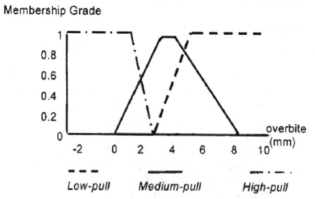

Fig. 26. Plot of membership functions for the input of overbite for each of three sets, . the low-, medium-, and high-pull types of headgear.

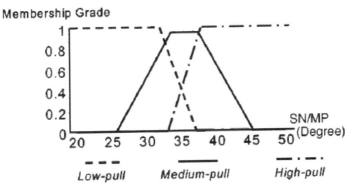

Fig. 27. Plot of membership functions for the input of mandibular for each of three sets, . the low-, medium-, and high-pull types of headgear.

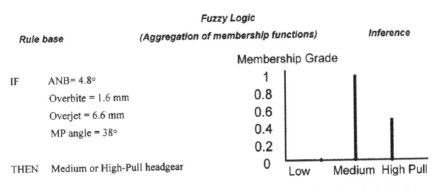

Fig. 28. The computer provides a selection of headgear types in which each choice is accompanied by a membership grades.

was the operation by multiple fuzzy sets were combined to produce single fuzzy set, the inference system was designed to calculate degrees of certainty for the use of each headgear type by means of membership grades fig 28.

The model was designed to calculate the degree of certainty for choosing low-, medium- or high-pull types of headgear. Eight orthodontic experts evaluated the decisions inferred by the system for 85 orthodontic cases. This group of clinicians was satisfied with the system's recommendations in 95.6 percent of the cases. In addition, the majority of the examiners (i.e. equal to or more than six out of eight) were satisfied with the system's recommendations in 97.6 per cent of the cases examined. Thus, the inference system developed was confirmed as being reliable and effective for clinical use in orthodontics.

4.3 The force system design for orthodontic treatments using AI

The most common aspects in the orthodontic treatment of extraction cases are the canine, the incisor and the mass retraction ,tooth retraction during space closure is achieved through two types of mechanics a. Sliding mechanics (friction mechanics) and b. Segmental or sectional mechanics (friction free technique). In the segmented arch technique, frictionless springs are used to attract the segments of teeth on either side of an attraction site , there are different retraction springs that can be used. Many variables affect the force system they could produce; geometry, material, cross section, position, activation distance, etc. Tooth movement and orthopedic changes are the result of an applied force system and the tissue response to it . The force system is currently the major factor that the orthodontist can control to achieve desirable orthodontic tooth movement. Force system generated from complex geometric appliances produce forces and moments, it's important to control not only the magnitude of the force but also the moment to force ratio to produce the desired tooth movement. Force systems originated from orthodontic appliances have been studied by means of static systems for simple springs[106,107]or by experimental method _[108-112], and numerical approaches _[113]_ or by dynamic systems (typodont systems) [114].The numerical methods are the most recent approaches having been merged with the medical area due to computer science, while in the experimental methods, the body of evidence is submitted to mechanical tests, which might determine the force system more accurately- [115]

During an orthodontic space closure, the optimum response, both clinically and histologically, depends on the precision and calibration of the force systems to be used, therefore; a variety of prefabricated and precalibrated orthodontic loops are able to deliver precise and carefully controlled forces was utilized. Attempts to improve the force systems produced by this appliance have resulted in a number of different loop designs. Control of the force systems applied to the teeth is one of the main challenges in orthodontic biomechanics. Thus, the theoretical prediction of the forces and moments produced by the orthodontic appliance is important to control treatment.

It can be seen that if a reliable analytical or numerical method of the closing loop analysis is available, then any orthodontist can use this tool to calculate the characteristics of the closing loops theoretically without resorting to costly and time-consuming experiments. In many previous studies many researchers were developed a mathematical models for simulating the force system produced by orthodontic appliances based on small-deflection linear theory, large-deflection nonlinear theory and finite element methods, the last decade witness the innovative AI modeling using soft computing approaches, The advantage for using a black box of AI elements (like Neural networks, Genetic algorithms) in simulating the force system produced by the orthodontic appliances its ability to capture the real behavior of the orthodontic appliances (spring system).

In this section we will discuss some of the available AI models that can be used in modeling of the effective design for appliances for orthodontic treatment.

5. Force system prediction using artificial neural network

As we mentioned above the retraction loops force system namely, force, moment and moment to force ratio is affected by various parameter, Kazem et al [116] produced an artificial neural network based on an experimental force system evaluation of T-retraction springs, the experimental procedure includes studying the effect of cross section and activation distance on the force system produced by T-retraction springs, Forty T-looped stainless steel arch wires of three different cross sections were used in the testing procedure ,their sizes were(0.018*0.025 in., 0.017*0.025 in., and 0.016*0.022 in.), A new test apparatus specially designed and operated by the researcher [117](Garma NMH) for the measurement of the horizontal forces and the moments of sectional springs is used for teeth retraction, Each one of the already prepared twenty sectional stainless steel T-loop of each group was activated by 1 mm, 2 mm, and 3 mm, respectively, and the readings from load cell outputs were recorded, .

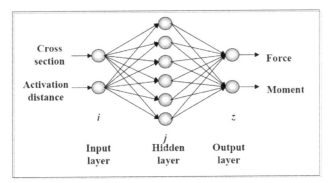

Fig. 29. NN architecture used for the force system modeling

After the results were obtained, they were used in the ANN modeling to evaluate its ability in the prediction process of the T-spring force system. Neural network training can be made more efficient if certain preprocessing steps are performed on the network inputs and targets. Figure 5 illustrates the preprocessing and postprocessing stage in prediction model. The neural network model is organized as a number of input neurons equal to the number of independent variables, which are spring properties (cross section and activation distance), and a number of output neurons equal to the number of dependent variable, which is the force system component (force and moment). Although the number of neurons in the input and output layers is specified depending on the problem, there is no hard and fast rules to specify the number of neurons in the hidden layer. Up to this day, the problem of specifying the optimal number of hidden neurons is an active area of research. Often a trial and error approach is starting with a modest number of hidden neurons and gradually increasing the number if the network fails to reduce its performance index (training error)[118,119]. The simulated annealing technique is used to capture the best weights and biases. The experimental results were used to train and test in neural network; seven measured results were used, from the total of nine, as data sets to train the network. Many neural networks architectures are used to train the data set to produce the least error; the neural network model was trained by using Levenberg - Marquardt Algorithm. many different trial numbers of the hidden layer neurons and types of the activation function were used at each time. Figure show optimized ANN training session. To evaluate the effect of increasing the hidden layer in to two layers on the ANN performance, many trial numbers of the two hidden layers training and accuracy prediction was done with different number of the two layer hidden neurons., the prediction accuracy for the testing patterns is based on the mean absolute percent error .

A network with one hidden layer include 6 neurons trained by Levenberg-Marquardt algorithm showed the best performance indication. Figure (20) shows the resulted network architecture, the network architecture consists of two input neurons (i), and one hidden layers contain six neuron (j) with nonlinear activation function (tangential sigmoid) and two output neurons (z) with linear activation function.

The prediction accuracy of the optimized ANN architecture are illustrated in (table), the mean error of data test set of the force prediction is (5.707%), while for the moment prediction is (4.048%),The multilayer feed forward neural network was successful in mapping the relationship among inputs parameters of the T-spring "cross section and activation distance" and output force system "horizontal force and moment." The successful ANN mapping of the relationship between the spring properties and resultant force system can happen by utilizing other researche\ results, and it would be more beneficial as generalization increased with increasing input data set _spring properties_ in this situation.

Set No.	Actual force (gm)	ANN Prediction	Error %	Moment (gm mm)	ANN Prediction	Error %
1	291.3	299.3	2.7487	1311.11	1301.7	0.7183`
8	375.3	342.8	8.666	2177.14	2016.5	7.3785

Table 3. Test data sets and network prediction after optimization

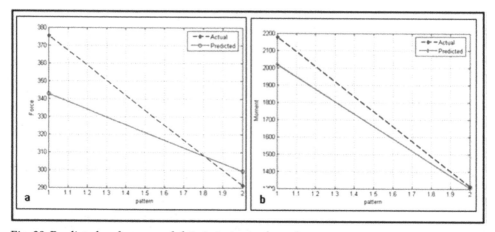

Fig. 30. Predicted and measured data in test set a-force, b- moment.

6. Multi-objective design optimization using GA

The multi-objective optimization is a vector of decision variables which satisfies constraints and optimizes vector functions whose elements represent the objective function. These functions form the mathematical description of performance criteria which are usually in conflict with each other. Hence, the term 'optimizes' means finding such a solution which would give the values of all objective functions acceptable to the designer, Osyczka [120].

The Genetic Algorithm is used in this work to optimize our engineering-orthodontic problem (select the best T-spring dimension and Material to get the required spring stiffness and moment to force ratio); i.e. to obtain an optimal force (spring stiffness) and a (M/H) ratio capable of pure translation together.

The spring design parameters are encoded directly, using real codification, as strings (chromosomes) to be used for GA. For T-spring thirteen parameters should be optimized as shown in the following chromosome:

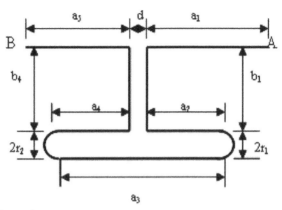

Fig. 31. T-spring Dimensions

$$x = [x_1 x_2, x_3, x_4, x_5, x_6, x_7, x_8, x_9, x_{10}, x_{11}, x_{12}, x_{13}] \qquad (2)$$

$$= [a_1, a_2, a_3, a_3, a_4, a_5, b_1, b_3, r_1,, r_2, d, t, w, E] \qquad (3)$$

Of these variables, a1, a2, a3, a4 ,a5,b1,b3, r1, r2 are real-parameters with specific range (Lmin, Lmax), t and w are discrete variables having the standard cross section dimensions values of orthodontic arch wires, E is a discrete variable having the standard Young's modulus values of orthodontic arch wires.

The two objective optimization problems are as follows [121]:

$$\text{Minimize } f_1(x) = springstiffness(kx) \quad \text{Minimize } f_2(x) = \|(M/H) - (M/H)_D\| \qquad (4)$$

Subjected to

$$g_1(x) = (x_1 + x_2 + x_3 + x_4 + x_5 + x_6 + x_7 + \pi x_8 + \pi x_9 + x_{10}) \ge (L_T)$$

$$g_4(x) = (x_1 + x_5 + x_{10}) \le (L_T)) \qquad (5)$$

$$g_2(x) = (x_6 + 2x_8) \le (H_T) \qquad (6)$$

$$g_3(x) = (x_7 + 2x_9) \le (H_T) \qquad (7)$$

$$g_5(x) = (x_2 + x_5 + x_{10}) \le (L_T)) \qquad (8)$$

$$g_6(x) = (x_2 + x_8 + x_9 + x_4) \le (x_1 + x_5 + x_{10}) \qquad (9)$$

$$g_7(x) = (x_3 + x_8 + x_9) \le (x_1 + x_5 + x_{10}) \qquad (10)$$

$$g_8(x) = x_2 + x_4 + x_{10} = x_3 \qquad (11)$$

$$g_9(x) = (x_6 + 2x_8) - (x_7 + 2x_9) \le \Delta \qquad (12)$$

Where the kx and M/H are calaculated using Castigliano's second theorem. (M/H)D is the required moment to force ratio for orthodontic treatment. The nine constraints are chosen to make sure that the produced solutions are within the required total spring dimensions (total length (LT) and total height (HT)). The maximum allowable difference in total height between the left and right end is given by (Δ). We can add any type of design constraint and to be sure that we will converge to some applicable design for the required application.

The presence or absence of a member in the spring structure is determined by comparing the length of the member with the designer defined small critical length, e. If a length is smaller than e, that member is assumed to be absent in the realized T-spring.

Operators in genetic algorithm

A new methodology for the optimization of the design parameters for T-spring arch wire had been developed by Kazem [121]. The proposed analytic model depending on the Castigliano's second theorem with an accurate boundary conditions and geometrical representation provides acceptable results for symmetric and asymmetric spring although it depends on the small deflection theory, in comparison with the results obtained using non-linear FEM. The multi-objective optimization for the spring design parameters is adopted successfully using GA method and the results show that depending on the above methodology, we can make good estimation of the required design parameters for the T-spring. Future work includes improving the analytical model for the spring system depending on the large deflection theorem and also, more inspection is needed by using other evolutionary algorithms like Strength Pareto Evolutionary Algorithm (SPEA) and SPEA 2 that update the ranking and selection criteria used in GA.

The initial population of strings (Real number coding) is generated at random and then the search is carried out among this population. The evolution of the population elements is non-generational, which means that the new replace the worst ones. The main different operators adopted in the GA are reproduction, crossover and mutation.

What concerns the reproduction operator is the successive generations of new strings which are generated based on their fitness values. In this case, a 5-tournament is used to select the strings for reproduction. For the tournament selection, only discrete values can be assigned and for higher range of selection intensity rather than ranking selection. About 50% of the population is lost at tournament size Tour=5. Tournament selection leads to high diversity for the same selection intensity compared to truncation selection [122]. At current search, tournament size less than 5 makes the solution progress slow toward the optimum solution and that which is more than 5 makes solution fall in the local optimum.

With a given probability Pc, the crossover operator adopts the single point technique and, therefore, the crossover point is only allowed between genes or, in other words, the crossover operator cannot disrupt genes. The mutation operator replaces one gene value xt with another one generated randomly with a specified range by a given probability Pm.

According to our knowledge, such an approach has not been tested yet on orthodontic spring optimum design problem.

The size of the mutation step is usually difficult to choose. The optimal step-size depends on the problem considered and may even vary during the optimization process. It is known, that small steps (small mutation steps) are often successful, especially when the individual is already well adapted. However, larger changes (large mutation steps) can, when successful, produce good results much quicker. Thus, a good mutation operator should often produce small step-sizes with a high probability and large step-sizes with a low probability.

Two indices are used to qualify the evolving solution. All indices are translated into penalty functions to be minimized. Each index is computed individually and is integrated in the fitness function evaluation. The fitness function ff adopted for evaluating the candidate solutions is defined after Coello and Christiansen [123]:

$$f_f = \beta_1 f_1 + \beta_2 f_2$$

Where $\beta_1 + \beta_2 = 1$

The optimization goal consists of finding a set of design parameters that minimize ff according to the priorities given by the weighting factors β_i (i = 1, 2), where each different set of weighting factors must result in a different solution.

Optimization weight factor (β_1, β_2)	Spring shape and material for Optimized solution vector (x)	f1			f2		
		GA	From FEM	Error %	GA	From FEM	Error%
(0.75,0.25)	txw=0.40x0.55 E=172,000Mpa	40.32	42.67	-5.8	1.31	1.11	15.2
(0.5,0.5)	txw=0.40x0.55 E=172,000Mpa	49.11	58.56	-19.2	1.66	1.4	15.6
(0.25,0.75)	txw=0.482x0.635 E=192,000Mpa	50.29	46.18	8.17	0.61	0.67	-9.8

Table 4. Optimized Solutions for T-Spring design.

The optimized spring geometry and materials produced by GA were modeled by using FEM to calculate the spring stiffness (=f1) and the difference between resultant moment to force ratio and the user specified ratio (=f2) as given in Table 4.

7. Summary

In summary the subject of artificial Intelligence (AI) deals with symbolic processing than numeric computation. Knowledge representation, reasoning, planning, learning, intelligent search and uncertainty management of data and knowledge are the common areas covered under AI. Some of the applications areas of AI are speech and image understanding, expert systems, pattern classification, system optimization and navigational planning of mobile robots, the recent implementation of AI in the medical field and orthodontics was of special concern in this chapter, as the discipline of orthodontics task is to deal with the boolean etiological identification and optimized strategies of solution delivered to treat dentoalveolar and/or facial skeletal malrelation, the AI role used to achieve this task using variant techniques , AI incorporated many trial of changing the techniques used to simulate the clinical situations in the three essential sequences, diagnosis, treatment plan and treatment. The presence of differential problematic orthodontic problems , their origins and the consequence treatment makes the understanding of the AI aspect and its techniques essential to choose the techniques discriminating different problems and subsequent solution. Three aspects of AI;

- Artificial Neural Nets
- Genetic Algorithms
- Fuzzy logic

Artificial intelligence trials with these three techniques in different orthodontic steps yield numerous researches enrich the orthodontic domain with logical and economic tool substitutes the elongated sequential and sophisticated techniques, these trials yet are active area of research and need elaborated studies to reach their ultimate clinical assumption.

8. References

[1] Konar A., Uncertainty Management in Expert Systems using Fuzzy Petri Nets, Ph.D. thesis, Jadavpur,1999.
[2] Newell, A .and Simon, H.A., Human Problem Solving, Prentice-Hall, Englewood Cliffs, NJ, 1972.
[3] Luger, G. F. and Stubblefield, W. A., Artificial Intelligence: Structures and Strategies for Complex Problem Solving, Benjamin/Cummings, Menlo Park, CA, 1993.
[4] Schalkoff, J., Culberson, J., Treloar, N. and Knight, B., "A world championship caliber checkers program," Artificial Intelligence, vol. 53, no. 2-3, pp. 273-289, 1992.
[5] Winston, P. H., Artificial Intelligence, Addison-Wesley, 2nd ed., Reading, MA, 1994.
[6] Newell, A .and Simon, H.A., Human Problem Solving, Prentice-Hall, Englewood Cliffs, NJ, 1972.
[7] Charniak, E. and McDermott, D., Introduction to Artificial Intelligence, Addison-Wesley, Reading, MA, 1985.
[8] E. A. Metzbower , J. J. DeLoach , "*Secondary effects in neural network analysis of the mechanical properties of welding alloys for HSLA shipbuilding steels*" Mathematical

Modeling of Weld Phenomena 6, eds H. Cerjak and H. K. D. H. Bhadeshia, published by Maney, London, 2002. pp. 231-242.

[9] H Demuth,M Beale,M Hagan "Neural Network Toolbox User's Guide Ver5 " the mathworks ,Inc.,Natick,MA,USA,2006

[10] D. T.Pham and L.Xing "Neural networks for identification, prediction and control" Springer publishing company (1997)

[11] Haykan Simon, "Neural Network – a comprehensive foundation", prentice Hall, 1999.

[12] Pohlheim, Hartmut, GEATbx: Introduction Evolutionary Algorithms: Overview, Methods and Operators GEATbx version 3.8 (2006)

[13] Zadeh L A 1965 Fuzzy sets. Information and Control 8: 338-353

[14] M. Hellmann, Fuzzy Logic Introduction Laboratoire Antennes Radar Telecom , F.R.E CNRS 2272, Equipe Radar Polarimetrie, Universit´e de Rennes, France

[15] Dean, T., Allen, J. and Aloimonds, Y., Artificial Intelligence: Theory and Practice, Addison-Wesley, Reading, MA, 1995.

[16] Dickmans, E.D., Mysliwetz, B. and Christians, T., "An integrated spatio-temporal approach to vehicles," IEEE Trans. on Systems, Man and Cybernetics, vol. 20, no. 6, Dec. 1990.

[17] Dougherty, E. R. and Giardina, C.R., Mathematical Methods for Artificial Intelligence and Autonomous Systems, Prentice-Hall, Englewood Cliffs, NJ, 1988.

[18] Feigenbaum, E. A. and Feldman, J., Eds., Computers and Thought, McGraw-Hill, New York, 1963.

[19] Haugeland, J., Ed., Artificial Intelligence: The Very Idea, MIT Press, Cambridge, 1985.

[20] Jackson, P., Introduction to Expert Systems, Addison-Wesley, Reading, MA, 1986.

[21] Hopfield JJ. Neural networks and physical systems with emergent collective computational abilities. Proc Nat Acad Sci. 1982; 2554- 2558.

[22] Kohonen T. Self-organised formation of topologically correct feature maps. Biological Cybernetics, 1982; 43: 59-69.

[23] Rummelhart DE, McLelland JL. Parallel distributed processing: Explorations in the microstructure of Cognition. Vol. I. Foundation, MIT Press 1987.

[24] Baxt, W. J., Application of artificial neural network to clinical medicine. Lancet. 346:1135–1138, 1995.

[25] Kocyigit, Y., Alkan, A., and Erol, H., Classification of EEG recordings by using fast independent component analysis and artificial neural network. J. Med. Syst. 32 (1)17–20, 2008.

[26] Silva Lopes H F & Abe J M. , Anghinah R. Application of Paraconsistent Artificial Neural Networks as a Method of Aid in the Diagnosis of Alzheimer Disease J Med Syst (2010) 34:1073–1081

[27] Ventouras, E. M., Monoyou, E. A., Ktonas, P. Y., Paparrigopoulos, T., Dikeos, D. G., Uzunoglu, N. K., and Soldatos, C. R., Sleep spindle detection using artificial neural networks trained with filtered timedomain EEG: a feasibility study. Comput. Methods Programs Biomed. 78 (3)191–207, 2005.

[28] Miller, A., The application of neural networks to imaging and signal processing in astronomy and medicine, Ph.D. thesis, Faculty of Science, Department of Physics, University of Southampton, 1993.

[29] Prado, J. C. A. Constelação fônica e redes neurais artificiais: aplicabilidade na análise computacional da produção da fala (in Portuguese). Ph.D. Thesis. FFLCH–USP; São Paulo, SP, BR; 2007.

[30] Weinstein, J., Kohn, K., and Grever, M., Neural computing in cancer drug development: predicting mechanism of action. Science. 258:447–451, 1992.

[31] Papik K, Molnar B, Schaefer R, Dombovari Z, Tulassay Z, Feher J. Application of neural network in medicine. Med Sci Monit. 1998; 4(3): 538-46.

[32] Sims-Williams J H, Brown I D, Matthewman A, Stephens C D 1987 A computer controlled expert system for orthodontic advice. British Dental Journal 163: 161-166

[33] Mackin N, Sims-Williams J H, Stephens C D 1991 Artificial intelligence in dental surgery: an orthodontic expert system, a dental tool of tomorrow. Dental Update 18: 341-343

[34] Hudson D L, Cohen M E 1994 Fuzzy logic in medical expert systems. IEEE Engineering in Medicine and Biology 3: 693-698

[35] Stephens C D, Mackin N, Sims-Williams J H 1996 The development and validation of an orthodontic expert system. British Journal of Orthodontics 23: 1-9

[36] Tanaka T, Miwa K, Kanda S 1997 Application of fuzzy reasoning in an expert system for ultrasonography. Dentomaxillofacial Radiology 26: 125-131

[37] Brown I D, Adams S R, Stephens C D, Erritt S J, Sims-Willianis J H 1991 The initial use of a computer controlled expert system in the treatment planning of Class II division 1 malocclusion. British Journal of Orthodontics 18: 1-7

[38] Graber TM, Vanarsdall RL. Orthodontics: Current principles and techniques. 2nd ed. St. Louis: Mosby, 1994.

[39] Xie X; Wang L; Wang A. Artificial Neural Network Modeling for Deciding if Extractions Are Necessary Prior to Orthodontic Treatment Angle Orthod. 2010;80:262–266.

[40] Stheeman S E, Van der Stelt P F, Mileman P A 1992 Expert systems in dentistry past performance—future prospects. Journal of Dentistry 20: 68-73

[41] Takada K, Sorihashi Y, Akcam M O 1998 Orthodontic treatment planning: its rationale for inference. In: Carels C, Willems G (eds) The future of orthodontics. Leuven University Press, Belgium, pp. 203-211

[42] Poon KC, Freer TJ. EICO-1: an orthodontist-maintained expert system in clinical orthodontics. Aust Orthod J. 1999; 15:219–228.

[43] Hammond RM, Freer TJ. Application of a case-based expert system to orthodontic diagnosis and treatment planning: a review of the literature. Aust Orthod J. 1996;14:150–153.

[44] Hammond RM, Freer TJ. Application of a case-based expert system to orthodontic diagnosis and treatment planning. Aust Orthod J. 1997;14:229–234.

[45] Lux CJ, Stellzig A, Volz D, Jäger W, Richardson A, Komposch G. Department of Orthodontics, Dental School, University of Heidelberg, Germany. Growh dev.aging. A neural network approach to the analysis and classification of human craniofacial growth. 1998:(6) 295-106

[46] Brickley MR, Shepherd JP, Armstrong RA. Neural networks: a new technique for development of decision support systems in dentistry. J Dent. 1998;26:305–309.

[47] S. Richmond, WC. Shaw, KD. O'Brien, IB. Buchanan, R. Jones ,CD. Stephens, CT. Roberts, M. Andrews, "The development of the par index (peer assessment rating): reliability and validity," European J of Orthodontics, vol. 14, no. 2, pp. 125-129, 1992.

[48] Zarei A, El-Sharkawi M, Hairfield M. An intelligent system for assessment of orthodontic treatment outcome using fuzzy union rule configuration. in Proc. IASTED, May 2007, 428-433.

[49] Zarei A, Hairfield M, Mirsaeidghazi SS. A Novel Neuro-Fuzzy Assessment Index for Orthodontics. IEEE Xplore. 2009;3493-3497.

[50] Vieira A, Lawrence H, Limeback H, Sampaio F, and Grynpas M. A visual analog scale for measuring dental fluorosis severity. American Dental Association, vol. 136, pp. 895-901, 2005.

[51] Takagi T and Sugeno M. Fuzzy identification of systems and its applications to modeling and control, IEEE Trans. Systems, Man. And Cybernetics, 1985;15: 116-132,.

[52] Jyh-Shing Roger Jang and Chuen-Tsai Sun, Neuro-fuzzy and control. in Proc. IEEE.1995; 83(3): 378-406.

[53] Cohen AM, Ip HH, Linney AD. A preliminary study of computer recognition and identification of skeletal landmarks as a new method of cephalometric analysis. Br J Orthod. 1984;

[54] Leonardi R, Giordano D, Maiorana F, Spampinato C. Automatic cephalometric analysis. Angle Orthod. 2008;78:145-15.

[55] Parthasarathy S, Nugent ST, Gregson PG, Fay DF. Automatic landmarking of cephalograms. Comput Biomed Res.1989;22:248–269.

[56] Tong W, Nugent ST, Jensen GM, Fay DF. An algorithm for locating landmarks on dental X-rays. Conference proceedings: 11th Annual International Conference of the IEEE Engineering in Medicine and Biology Society. IEEE 1989(2): 552–554.

[57] Forsyth DB, Davis DN. Assessment of an automated cephalometric analysis system. Eur J Orthod. 1996;18:471–478.

[58] Ren J, Lid D, Feng D, Shao J. A knowledge-based automatic cephalometric analysis method. Conference proceedings: 20th International Conference of the IEEE Engineering in Medicine and Biology Society. IEEE 1998;20(2):723–727.

[59] Cardillo J, Sid-Ahmed MA. An image processing system for locating craniofacial landmarks. IEEE T Med Imaging. 1994; 13:275–289.

[60] Rudolph DJ, Sinclair PM, Coggins JM. Automatic computerized radiographic identification of cephalometric landmarks. Am J Orthod Dentofacial Orthop. 1998;113:173– 179.

[61] Hutton TJ, Cunningham S, Hammond P. An evaluation of active shape models for the automatic identification of cephalometric landmarks. Eur J Orthod. 2000;22:499–508.

[62] Romaniuk B, Desvignes M, Revenu M, Deshayes MJ. Shape variability and spatial relationships modeling in statistical pattern recognition. Pattern Recogn Lett. 2004;25: 239–247.

[63] Saad AA, El-Bialy A, Kandil AH, Sayed AA. Automatic cephalometric analysis using active appearance model and simulated annealing. GVIP 05. Conference proceedings: InterAUTOMATIC

[64] CEPHALOMETRIC ANALYSIS 151 Angle Orthodontist, Vol 78, No 1, 2008 national Conference on Graphics, Vision and Image Processing, 2005 Dec 19-21, Cairo, Egypt (2005). ICGST; 2005.

[65] Innes A, Ciesielski V, Mamutil J, Sabu J. Landmark detection for cephalometric radiology images using pulse coupled neural networks. In: Arabnia H, Mun Y, eds. Conference proceedings: IC-AI '02, International Conference on Artificial Intelligence, 2002 June 24–27, Las Vegas, Nevada. CSREA Press; 2002;2:511–517.

[66] Chakrabartty S, Yagi M, Shibata T, Cauwenberghs G. Robust cephalometric identification using support vector machines. Conference proceedings: ICME '03,

International Conference on Multimedia and Expo, 2003 Jul 6–9. IEEE 2003;III:429–432. 32.

[67] Ciesielski V, Innes A, Sabu J, Mamutil J. Genetic programming for landmark detection in cephalometric radiology images. Int J Knowl Based Intell Eng Syst. 2003;7:164–171.

[68] El-Feghi I, Sid-Ahmed MA, Ahmadi M. Automatic localization of craniofacial landmarks for assisted cephalometry. Pattern Recognit. 2004;37:609–621.

[69] Liu J, Chen Y, Cheng K. Accuracy of computerized automatic identification of cephalometric landmarks. Am J Orthod Dentofacial Orthop. 2000;118:535–540.

[70] Grau V, Alcaniz M, Juan MC, Monserrat C, Knoll C. Automatic localization of cephalometric landmarks. J Biomed Inform. 2001;34:146–156. 34.

[71] Yang J, Ling X, Lu Y, Wei M, Ding G. Cephalometric image analysis and measurement for orthognathic surgery. Med Biol Eng Comput. 2001;39:279–284.

[72] Giordano D, Leonardi R, Maiorana F, Cristaldi G, Distefano M. Automatic landmarking of cephalograms by CNNS. Lect Notes Artif Int. 2005;3581:342–352.

[73] Yue W, Yin D, Li C, Wang G, Xu T. Automated 2-D cephalometric analysis on X-ray images by a model-based approach. IEEE Trans Biomed Eng. 2006;53:1615–1623.

[74] Abe JM. Paraconsistent Artificial Neural Networks: an Introduction, Lecture Notes in Artificial Intelligence. Carbonell & J. Siekmann, 2004.

[75] Mario M C, Abe J M., Ortega N R S., Santo Jr M D. Paraconsistent Artificial Neural Network as Auxiliary in Cephalometric Diagnosis. Artificial Organs2010 34(7):E215–E221,Wiley Periodicals, Inc..

[76] Sylvan R, Abe JM. On general annotated logics, with an introduction to full accounting logics. Bull Symb Log 1996;2:118–9.

[77] Mario MC. Modelo de análise de variáveis craniométricas através das Redes Neurais Artificiais Paraconsistentes. PhD thesis, University of São Paulo, 2006.

[78] Da Silva Filho JI, Abe JM. Fundamentos das Redes Neurais Paraconsistentes – Destacando Aplicações em Neurocomputação, (in Portuguese) Editôra Arte & Ciência: ISBN 85-7473-045-9. 2001;247.

[79] Ricketts RM. Cephalometric analysis and synthesis. AngleOrthod 1961;31:141–56.

[80] Tanikawa C, Yagi M, Takada K. Automated Cephalometry: System Performance Reliability Using Landmark-Dependent Criteria. Angle Orthod. 2009;79:1037–1046.

[81] Shibata T. Intelligent VLSI systems based on a psychologicalbrain model. Proc IEEE Int Sym on Intelligent Signal

[82] Yagi M, Shibata T. An image representation algorithm compatible to neural-associative-processor-based hardware recognition systems. IEEE Trans Neural Netw. 2003;14(5):1144–1161.

[83] Levy-Mandel AD, Venetsanopoulos AN, Tsotsos JK. Knowledge- based landmarking of cephalograms. Comput Biomed Res. 1986;282–309.

[84] Takada K, Yagi M, Tanikawa C. Dependable systems for decisions in clinical dentistry-how electronics implements what dentists know. Proc Int Sym on Advanced Electronics for Future Generations, "Secure-Life Electronics" for Quality Life and Society. 2005 Oct 11–12, Tokyo, Japan. 2005:15– 21.

[85] Baumrind S, Frantz RC. The reliability of head film measurements. 1. Landmark identification. Am J Orthod. 1971; 60:111–127

[86] Fujita K, Takada K, QianRong G, Shibata T. Patterning of human dental arch wire blanks using a vector quantization algorithm. Angle Orthod. 2002;72:285–294.

[87] Levy-Mandel AD, Venetsanopoulos AN, Tsotsos JK. Knowledge- based landmarking of cephalograms. Comput Biomed Res. 1986;282–309.

[88] Rudolph DJ, Sinclair PM, Coggins JM. Automatic computerized radiographic identification of cephalometric landmarks. Am J Orthod Dentofacial Orthop. 1998;113:173– 179.

[89] Romaniuk B, Desvignes M, Revenu M, Deshayes MJ. Shape variability and spatial relationships modeling in statistical patter recognition. Pattern Recogn Lett. 2004;25: 239–247.

[90] Grau V, Alcaniz M, Juan MC, Monserra C, Knoll C. Automatic localization of cephalometric landmarks. J Biomed Inform. 2001;34:146–156.

[91] Ciesielski V, Innes A, Mamutil J. Genetic programming for landmark detection in cephalometric radiology images. Int J Knowl Base Intell Eng Syst. 2003;7:164–171.

[92] Giordano D, Leonardi R, Maiorana F, Cristaldi G, Distefano ML. Automatic landmarking of cephalograms by cellular neural networks. Lect Notes Artif Int. 2005;3581:342–352.

[93] Yue W, Yin D, Wang G, Xu T. Automated 2-D cephalometric analysis on X-ray images by a model-based approach. IEEE Trans Biomedical Eng. 2006;53:1615–1623.

[94] Banumathi A, Raju S. , Abhaikumar V. Diagnosis of Dental Deformities in Cephalometry Images Using Support Vector Machine J Med Syst (2011) 35:113–119

[95] Romaniuk, B., Desvignes, M., Robiaille, J., Revenu, M., Deshayes, M. J., Augmented reality and semi automated landmarking of cephalometry radiographs. Comput. Anal. Images Patterns, 9th International Conference CAIP 2001. 410–418, 2001. Sep 5-7

[96] Ericson S, Kurol J. Radiographic assessment of maxillary canine eruption in children with clinical signs of eruption disturbance. Eur J Orthod 1986;8:133-40.

[97] Ericson S, Kurol J. Early treatment of palatally erupting maxillary canines by extraction of the primary canines. Eur J Orthod 1988; 10:283-95.

[98] Stewart JA, Heo G, Giover KE, Williamson PC, Lam EWN, Major PW. Factors that relate to treatment duration for patients with palatally impacted maxillary canines. Am J Orthod Dentofacial Orthop 2001;119:216-25.

[99] Crescini A, Nieri M, Buti J, Baccetti T, Mauro S, Pini Prato GP. Short- and long-term periodontal evaluation of impacted canines treated with a closed surgical-orthodontic approach. J Clin Periodontol 2007;34:232-42.

[100] Crescini A, Nieri M, Buti J, Baccetti T, Pini Prato GP. Pre-treatment radiographic features for the periodontal prognosis of treated impacted canines. J Clin Periodontol 2007;34:581-7.

[101] Nieri M, Crescini A, Rotundo R, Baccetti T, C Pierpaolo, Pratoe GPP. Factors affecting the clinical approach to impacted maxillary canines: A Bayesian network analysis. Am J Orthod Dentofacial Orthop 2010;137:755-62.

[102] Crescini A, Nieri M, Buti J, Baccetti T, Pini Prato GP. Orthodontic and periodontal outcomes of treated impacted maxillary canines. Angle Orthod 2007;77:571-7.

[103] Proffit W R, Fields H W, Sarver DM,Contemporary orthodontics. Mosby Elsevier,4th ed., 2007.

[104] Akgam M. O, Takada K. Fuzzy modelling for selecting headgear types. European Journal of Orthodontics.2002(24):99-106.

[105] Williams J K, Cook P A, Isaacson K G, Thorn A R Fixed orthodontic appliances — principles and practice.1996, Wright, Oxford

[106] Braun, S., and Garcia, J. L., 2002, "The Gable Bend Revisited," Am. J. Orthod. Dentofacial Orthop., 122, pp. 523–527.

[107] Choy, K., Pae, E., Park, Y. C., and Burstone, C. J., 2002, "Controlled Space Closure With Statically Determinate Retraction System," Angle Orthod., 72, pp. 191–198.

[108] Solonche, D. J., Burstone, C. J., and Vanderby, R., 1977, "A Device for Determining the Mechanical Behavior of Orthodontic Appliances," IEEE Trans. Biomed. Eng., BME-24, pp. 538–539.

[109] Nagerl, H., Burstone, C. J., Beacher, B., and Messenburg, D. K., 1991, "Center of Rotation With Transverse Forces," Am. J. Orthod. Dentofacial Orthop., 99, pp. 337–345.

[110] Braun, S., Sjursen, R. C., and Legan, H. L., 1997, "On the Management of Extraction Sites," Am. J. Orthod. Dentofacial Orthop., 112, pp. 645–655.

[111] Siatkowski, R. E., 1997, "Continuous Arch Wire Closing Loop Design, optimization, and Verification Part I," Am. J. Orthod. Dentofacial Orthop., 112, pp. 393–402.

[112] Ferreira, M. A., 1999, "The Wire Material and Cross Section Effect on Double Delta Closing Loops Regarding Load and Spring Rate Magnitude: An In Vitro Study," Am. J. Orthod. Dentofacial Orthop., 115, pp. 275–282.

[113] Raboud, D. W., Faulkner, M. G., Lipsett, A. W., and Haberstock, D. L., 1997,"Three Dimensional Effects in Retraction Appliance Design," Am. J. Orthod. Dentofacial Orthop., 112, pp. 378–392.

[114] Rhee, J., Chu, Y., and Row, J., 2001, "A Comparison Between Friction and Frictionless Mechanics With a New Type Simulation System," Am. J. Orthod. Dentofacial Orthop., 119, pp. 292–299.

[115] Ferreira, M. A., Oliveira, F. T., Ignacio, S. A., and Borges, P. C., 2005, Experimental Force Definition System for a New Orthodontic Retraction Spring," Angle Orthod., 75_3_, pp. 368–377.

[116] Kazem B. I, ; Ghaib N. H;. Garma N. M. H., "Experimental Investigation and Neural Network Modeling for Force System of Retraction T-Spring for Orthodontic Treatment"; Journal of Medical Devices ,ASME, Vol 4, 2010, pp 021001-1-7.,

[117] Garma N. M. H., An experimental and artificial neural network prediction of cross section and activation distance effect on T-spring force system. Master's thesis. Department of orthodontics, Baghdad.

[118] Sukthomya, W., and Tannock, J., 2005, "The Training of Neural Networks to Model Manufacturing Processes," J. Intell. Manuf., 16_1_, pp. 39–51.

[119] Yousif, K. Y., Daws, K. M., and Kazem, B. I., 2008, "Prediction of Friction stir welding Characteristics Using Neural Network," Jordan Journal of Mechanical and Industrial Engineering _JJMIE_, 2_3_, pp. 151–155.

[120] Osyczka, A., 1985, "Multicriteria Optimization for Engineering Design," in Design Optimization, J. S. Gero, ed., Academic, New York, pp. 193–227.

[121] Bahaa I Kazem "Multi-Objective Optimization for the Force System of Orthodontic Retraction Spring Using Genetic Algorithms ";Journal of Medical Devices ,ASME, Vol 3, 2009, pp 041006-1-7.,

[122] Pohlheim, H., 2004, "GEATbx Introduction Evolutionary Algorithms: Overview, Methods and Operators," Version 3.5a, July 2004, http:// www.geatbx.com

[123] Coello, C. A., and Christiansen, A. D., 2000, "Multiobjective Optimization for Trusses Using Genetic Algorithms," Comput. Struct., 75, pp. 647–660.

9

Clinical Application of Three-Dimensional Reverse Engineering Technology in Orthodontic Diagnosis

Bong-Kuen Cha
Gangneung-Wonju National University
Korea

1. Introduction

A three-dimensional (3D) surface scanning system was recently introduced in dental fields and has been used most extensively for example, for assessing morphological changes in maxillofacial surgery or in orthopedic treatment with a functional appliance. Another use for the 3D data acquisition in orthodontics is bending art system (BAS) or Invisalign® system introduced as a new treatment modality. However, research on the various clinical applications of 3D digital model is still in its early stage, as it has been used as a simple model analysis, a digitized data storage (Alcan *et al.*, 2009; Ayoub *et al.*, 2003; Birnbaum & Aaronson, 2008; Cha *et al.*, 2007; Choi et al., 2010; Costalos *et al.*, 2005; Dalstra & Melsen, 2009; Gracco *et al.*, 2007; Keating *et al.*, 2008; Krejci *et al.*, 1994; Leifert *et al.*, 2009; Macchi et al., 2006; Santoro *et al.*, 2003; Stevens *et al.*, 2006; Van der Linden, 1987).

This chapter is intended to investigate the possibility of the clinical application of 3D reverse engineering technology used in the analysis of orthodontic models and facial morphology.

The theme of this chapter is divided into seven parts:

1. The measuring accuracy and process of the 3D model scanning technique was evaluated in terms of linear, surface and volumetric parameters. The diverse clinical applications of model analysis, including measuring basal arch width, or sectional areas concerned will be presented.
2. Giving the evidences that the superimposition of the 3D digital maxillary model is clinically as reliable as cephalometric superimposition for assessing orthodontic tooth movements.
3. Presenting the clinical cases, using the superimposition technique for the 3D measuring of orthodontic tooth movement in maxilla.
4. Describing the clinical procedure for digital diagnostic setup.
5. Introducing a novel method concerning the volumetric assessment of tooth wear using 3D reverse engineering technology.
6. Presenting a quantitative 3D soft tissue facial analysis using a color coding system.
7. Presenting feasible methods of the integrating 3D digital model into a 3D facial image to visualize the anatomic position of the dentition.

1.1 Reliability of measurement and clinical application of 3D digital model

The accuracy and reproducibility of a 3D surface scanning device to record the surface detail of study models is well documented and evaluated with respect to linear, surface, and volumetric parameters in the literature (Alcan *et al.*, 2009; Cha *et al.*, 2007; Costalos *et al.*, 2005; Dalstra & Melsen, 2009; Eraso et al., 2007; Gracco et al., 2007; Horton et al., 2009; Keating *et al.*, 2008; Leifert *et al.*, 2009; Miller et al., 2003). We have taken a comparison study using 30 dental study models (Cha et al., 2007). Orthodontic linear measurements were recorded between landmarks, directly on the study models and indirectly on the 3D digital models by using the INUS dental scanning solution® (composed of Breuckmann's opto TOP scanner®, INUS Rapidform 2002®, Autoscan system®). The resolution of the Topometric & Photogrametric 3D scanner® after calibration is 8 μm and the reliability is 15 μm. This exceeds the accuracy required for orthodontic measurements such as the mesiodistal tooth width, arch length, and arch width. There were no significant differences between the measurements at the 1% level. The similar study (Keating et al., 2008) using another laser scanning device (Minolta VIVID® 900, non-contact 3D surface laser scanner, Konica Minolta Inc., Tokyo, Japan) also shows that the difference between measurements on the study and 3D digital models was 0.14 mm, and was not statistically significant. In conclusion, measurements carried out on 3D digital models are a valid and reliable alternative to those currently used in study models in orthodontic practice with the advantage of significantly reducing measurement time.

1.2 Some examples of research and clinical applications using 3D digital model

Tooth size, crowding or spacing, overjet, overbite, and Bolton analysis are typically measured by hand on study models. 3D digital model is valuable alternative to conventional study models and can be used to determine routine diagnostic value, such as the Bolton analysis, arch length discrepancy, sagittal or transverse symmetry (Cha et al., 2007; Santoro et al., 2003) (Fig. 1). Automatic identification system (the automatic recognition of tooth morphology) will be a suite of technologies, that enable and facilitate the accurate capture and rapid transmission of machine readable data, e.g. cusp tip or pit and fissure of certain teeth, to automated information systems, thereby enhancing the readiness of capabilities in support of their respective mission.

Furthermore it also held information, which could previously be gathered only by complicated laboratory procedure, as sawing or wax up etc. There are numerous clinical examples to illustrate how such information could be applied in the diagnostic or treatment evaluation in orthodontics (Fig. 2). In counterpoint to the two-dimensional analysis, it is possible with 3D digital model to determine further parameters, such as palatal volume before and after maxillary expansion (Fig. 3) or volume or surface square measure of the deep structure of the palate (Fig. 4).

3D digital model offers many advantages, including elimination of model breakage and storage problems, instant retrieval of models, ease of communication with patients and colleagues. A single set of 3D digital models typically requires 8 MByte of disc space. It means that the data of 5,000 patients can be stored on a 40 GByte drive. It enables the orthodontist to e-mail images if desired and is a convenient presentation tool (Cha *et al.*, 2007).

Disadvantages include lack of tactile input for the orthodontist and time needed to learn how to use the system (Santoro *et al.*, 2003). 3D digital models present several unique challenges compared with conventional study models. Because the 3D computer image is

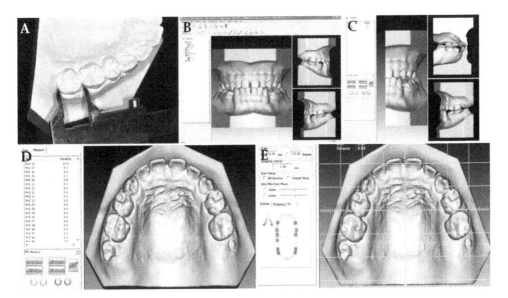

Fig. 1. **A**. Tooth size analysis: traditional manual method with sliding caliper. **B**. Gallery 3D digital model images in 3Txer software®(Orapix Co., Seoul, Korea). **C**. Selection of digital model for overbite and overjet measurements. Models can be rotated, which facilitates cross-sectioning at point of maximum overjet. **D**. Tooth size measurement tools (mesiodistal diameters) in 3Txer software®. **E**. Assessment of sagittal and transverse arch form symmetry in 3Txer software®.

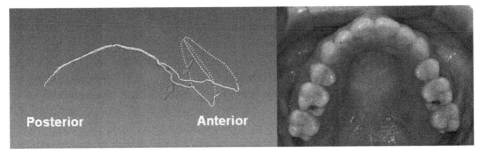

Fig. 2. Notice the change in palatal surface with gingival enlargement after retraction of anterior teeth. Enlarged soft tissue was denoted by the red arrow.

displayed on a 2D screen, the greatest challenge was observing crossbite. They will seem to have a positive overjet in the posterior segment when they really do not. Details for midlines, occlusal anatomy, and wear facets are not as clear on the 3D digital model (Stevens *et al.*, 2006).

Despite such limitations, 3D digital model provide a valuable source of information and continuous development of technology will suggest ways to overcome some of its shortcomings.

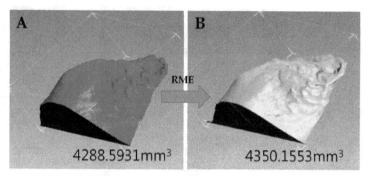

Fig. 3. Volumetric change of the palate before **A** and after **B** rapid maxillary expansion (volumetric change was about 61.6 mm³).

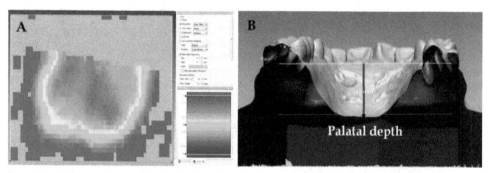

Fig. 4. **A.** Color contour analysis locating the deepest point that cannot be recognized accurately by manual method, light green means zero point, dark red area means deepest point of palate. **B.** Measuring accurate palatal depth from the arbitrary reference plane to the deepest point of mid-palatal suture located by using color contour analysis.

2. Evidences that the superimposition of the 3D digital maxillary model is clinically as reliable as cephalometric superimposition for assessing orthodontic tooth movement

Despite inherent errors, cephalometric superimpositions are currently the most widely used means for assessing sagittal and vertical tooth movement. However, there are some disadvantages and limitations of cephalometric radiographs and superimposition. Its drawbacks include difficulties in evaluating 3D tooth movement and identifying inherent landmarks. Further disadvantages are tracing errors, frequent radiation exposure, and high costs (Ghafari *et al.*, 1998).

We have performed a study, comparing 3D digital model superimposition with cephalometric superimposition (Cha *et al.*, 2007). The material was collected from initial and final maxillary study models and lateral cephalometric radiographs of 30 patients, who underwent orthodontic treatment with extraction of permanent teeth. The 3D superimposition was carried out using the surface-to-surface matching (best-fit method)

(Fig. 5). The antero-posterior movement of the maxillary first molar and central incisor was evaluated cephalometrically and on 3D digital models. The results revealed no statistical differences between the incisor and molar movements as assessed cephalometrically and by 3D model superimposition. These findings suggest that the 3D digital model superimposition technique used in this study is clinically as reliable as cephalometric superimposition for assessing orthodontic tooth movements.

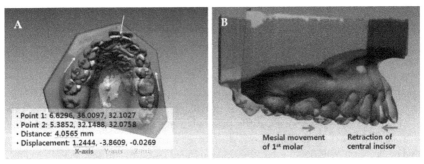

Fig. 5. Assessment of tooth movements on superimposed 3D digital models (red: before treatment, blue: after treatment). A. Occlusal view. B. Sagittal view.

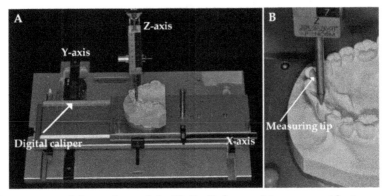

Fig. 6. Measurement of the study model with the Reference Measurement Instrument (RMI) A. Digital calipers for X-, Y-, and Z-axis. B. Measuring from the tip of the canine.

To evaluate the accuracy of the superimposition of 3D digital models using the palatal surface as a reference for measuring tooth movements, we have performed a comparison study of the correlation between the tooth movement of the setup model and that of the superimposition in its 3D digital model (Choi et al., 2010). Teeth on the study model were randomly moved after sawing, subsequently scanned to produce another set of 3D digital models. 3D digital model were superimposed using the palatal area as reference via surface-to-surface matching and the changes in tooth movement were calculated. In the study models, the tooth movements were directly measured using the Reference Measurement Instrument (Fig. 6). The means of the anteroposterior (x-axis), transverse (y-axis), and vertical (z-axis) tooth movements of the study models and those of the digital models did not differ significantly, and very high correlations were found between the study models and the digital models.

Recently, Jang et al. (Jang et al., 2009) superimposed serial models treated by premolar extraction by means of three miniscrews as registration landmarks (miniscrew-superimposition method) and compared with ruga-palate superimposition method. The displacement of the central incisors measured using the ruga-palate-superimposition method showed no significant difference with that measured using the miniscrew-superimposition method.

Moreover, with the superimposition method introduced here, it seems promising that, in the future, a simple mouse click will enable fast computer-assisted evaluation of 3D tooth movements (Choi et al., 2010).

Despite promising possibilities of the applications, the validity of this method has not been examined in growing patients, who underwent orthopedic treatment, such as rapid maxillary expansion (RME) treatment or maxillary surgery. In addition, we must not overlook the fact, that we encounter difficulties when we try to superimpose the mandibular arch because of the lack of the stable registration area (Fig. 7). Further research on this field is needed to clarify the evidences for the stable area for the superimposition.

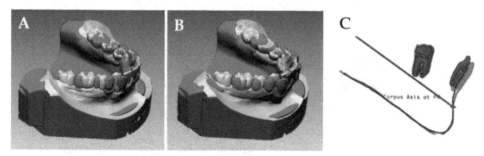

Fig. 7. Different results of mandibular superimposition due to the lack of stable registration area. Superimposition (**A**) shows no lingual movement of lower incisor. Note the tremendous lingual movement of lower incisor on superimposition (**B**) in same patient (red: before treatment, blue: after treatment). C. Superimposition on mandible in 2D cephalometrics shows lingual movement of lower incisor.

3. Presentation of clinical cases, using the superimposition technique for the 3D measurement of orthodontic tooth movement in maxilla

A 32-year-old Korean female presented with chief complaint of facial convexity. Cephalometric analysis showed a skeletal Class II relationship, significant obtuse mandibular plane angle, and retrognathic chin. After extraction of four premolars, pre-adjusted fixed appliances were bonded for initial leveling and alignment of both arches. An L-shaped mini-plate was adjusted to fit the contour of each cortical bone surface and was fixed with bone screws with the long arm exposed to the oral cavity, between upper first and second molars, for the intrusion of upper molars and retraction of upper dentition without any anchorage loss. After 30 months of orthodontic treatment, the patient showed a Class I occlusion with normal overbite, overjet and improved profile (Fig. 8).

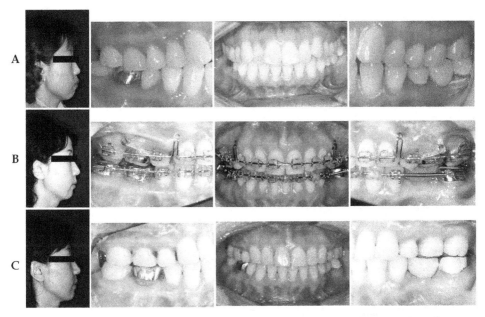

Fig. 8. A 32-year-old female with skeletal Class II relatiohship, hyperdivergent long-face pattern, and retrognathic chin. **A**. Pre-treatment. **B**. Contraction arch and miniplate for retraction of anterior teeth and intrusion of posterior teeth. **C**. Post-treatment.

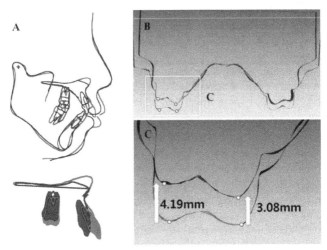

Fig. 9. **A**. Superimposition of pre-and post-treatment cephalometric tracings. Significant intrusion and distalization of upper molars were noted. (red: before treatment, blue: after treatment) **B**. Superimposition using 3D digital models. **C**. The amount of intrusion on the buccal and palatal cusp can be measured on the superimposed 3D digital models respectively. Note the different amount of intrusion between buccal and palatal cusp.

Superimposition of the pre- and post-treatment cephalometric radiography demonstrated significant intrusion of the upper posterior teeth. The entire upper dentition appeared to have been retracted. Fig. 9 shows, that in superimposed 3D digital model between before and after orthodontic treatment, the mesiobuccal cusp of upper right first molar was intruded 4.2 mm, on the other hand, palatal cusp as a functional cusp, was intruded only 3.1 mm. Such a result, it is impossible for us to get with the conventional cephalometric superimposition method.

A 10-year-old girl presented with a skeletal Class III malocclusion, a concave facial profile due to an anterior crossbite. Based on the cephalometric and clinical examinations, the patient was diagnosed as a functional Class III. The treatment plan for this patient included Class III activator (Fig. 10).

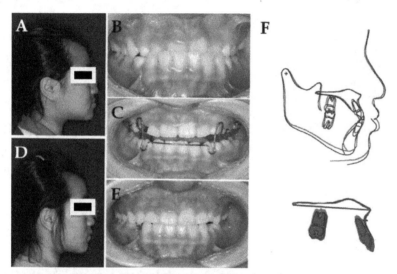

Fig. 10. A, B. Pre-treatment. Notice the anterior crossbite. C. Class III activator was used. D, E. Post-treatment. Notice normal overjet and overbite. F. Superimposition of pre-and post-treatment shows extrusion of upper molar and labioversion of upper incisors. (red: before treatment, blue: after treatment)

Post-treatment superimposed tracing revealed that anterior crossbite was corrected mainly by dentoalveolar movement and clockwise rotation of the mandible (Fig. 10). The maxillary incisors were flared and mandibular incisors were retruded and somehow extruded. However, correct measurement of the amount of tooth movement was not possible, because of inherent errors of the tracing and bisecting tracing of the cephalometrics.

The extrusion of upper molars exerts a downward vector of force on the mandible, causing the lower jaw to rotate downwards and backwards in a clockwise direction. Palatal cusp specially plays a more important role in this phenomenon rather than buccal cusp, which we are unable to measure separately in conventional superimposition of the 2D cephalometrics. Fig. 11 shows, that in superimposed 3D digital model between before and after orthodontic treatment, the mesiobuccal cusp of right upper first molar extruded 2.21 mm, on the other hand, mesiopalatal cusp as a functional cusp, extruded 1.30 mm. This different result might come from the change of the amount in the torque of the upper molars

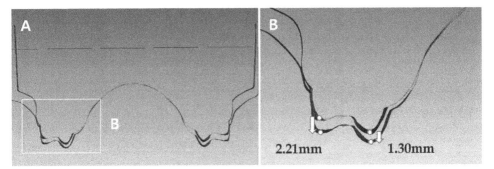

Fig. 11. **A, B** Different amount of the extrusion between mesiobuccal cusp and mesiopalatal cusp, which plays an important role as a functional cusp.

4. The clinical procedure for digital diagnostic setup and fabrication of indirect bonding tray

The diagnostic setup is a valuable aid in testing the effect of complex therapy, such as asymmetric extractions, space redistribution in the congenital missing cases. By replacing the teeth on the model in their desired position after suitable trimming, one can obtain an idea of the proportions between dental arch, apical area, occlusion and the degree to which the anterior teeth should be displaced sagittally (Fig. 12)(Van der Linden, 1987). The infusion of computer-aided design/computer-assisted machining (CAD/CAM Technology) enables now orthodontist or technicians to make virtual diagnostic setup, that provide not only diagnostic aids, but also simplify the laboratory procedure for precise indirect bonding (Fig. 13).

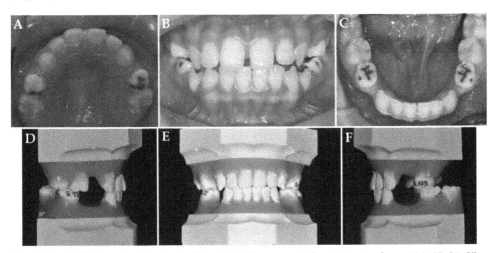

Fig. 12. **A~C.** This patient is Angle Class III with congenital missing teeth on #14, 15, 24, 25, 34, 35, 44, and 45. Treatment planning is prosthodontic treatment for #15, 25, 34, 35, 44, and 45 with full protraction of maxillary buccal teeth, as the lower anterior group remains unchanged. **D~F.** Traditional diagnostic set-up model.

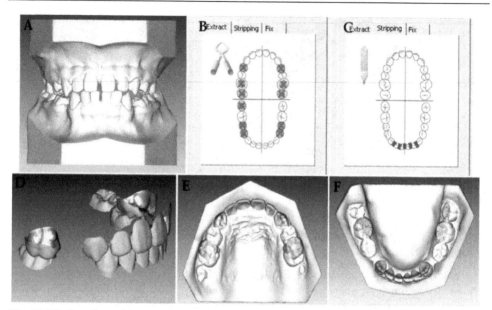

Fig. 13. 3D digital model in 3Txer software® (Orapix Co., Seoul, Korea). A~C. The program includes extractions or stripping functions, which can be planned in diagnostic set-up. In this case, we use "Extract" function. D. 3D virtual set-up in 3Txer software®. E, F. Superimpositions before and after set-up can visualize and quantify tooth movement in comparison to traditional set-up.

It is important in making the diagnostic setup to select correct arch form. For this purpose, we use an individualized template, which is able to give the precise arch form for each patient, provided by the 3Txer software® (Orapix Co., Seoul, Korea). These references are selected by the practitioner from a 3D virtual setup with virtual bracket positioning (Fig. 13).

Bracket positioning is an important factor for efficient orthodontic treatment. Traditionally, direct bonding of the bracket is used by most of the orthodontists. Advantages of direct bonding over the indirect procedure were summarized as follows (Zachrisson & Brobakken, 1978);

1.   The bracket bases were fitted closer to the tooth surface.
2.   It was easier to remove excess adhesive flash around the bracket bases.
3.   The bonding adhesive constantly filled out the entire contact surface of the bracket.

As straight arch wire technique and lingual orthodontics were developed, because of the irregularity of lingual or labial tooth surface and the difficulty of access to some teeth, indirect bonding became very rapidly the technique of choice (Fillion, 2007).

Indirect bonding technique may be classified into two main categories; procedure with, or without setup of individual teeth. The difference between the two procedures is that while the purpose of the indirect bonding without setup is to reduce the possible positioning error often confronted in direct bonding, with setup is to realize the ideal straight arch wire technique that does not require arch wire bending. Fig. 14 shows typical procedure of indirect bonding without setup, using dual tray method.

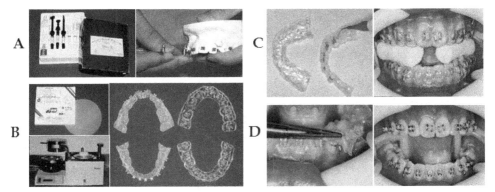

Fig. 14. Indirect bonding procedure. **A.** Apply double coat of liquid separator to dry stone models and positioning brackets using Phase II composite® on brackets' base. **B.** Fabricate two indirect transfer trays using 0.5 mm Copyplast material and 1.25 mm Biocryl material from Bioplast® company. **C.** Brackets' base is rinsed with acetone and the teeth are etched, rinsed, and dried. Excel composite® is added to brackets' base and the dual trays are applied. **D.** Removing transfer trays.

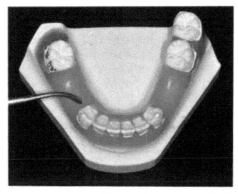

Fig. 15. The individual teeth are sawn out. Setting the separate block on the wax roll permits alternations in position.

In 1982, Myrberg and Warner (Myrberg & Warner, 1982) presented a technique, in which individual bracket placement indicators were made for each tooth based on the concept of a dental setup that suits the individual functional, occlusal, and esthetic requirements of each patient. Subsequent to this, numerous techniques have been developed based on indirect bonding from diagnostic setups (Hoffman, 1988). The traditional method of fabricating a diagnostic setup is to saw through the root areas, separate the teeth by hand, and affix them in their new positions with wax (Fig. 15). The technique is difficult to master and furthermore the laboratory procedure is tedious and time consuming for both the technician and orthodontist.

The rapid development of CAD/CAM technology enables not only bonding the brackets in preciously corrected position, but ensures that their individualized placements will produce the ideal occlusion incorporated in the virtual setup (Fillion, 2007).

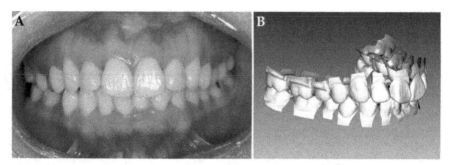

Fig. 16. **A**. This patient's chief complaint was anterior crowding. **B**. Visualization of the scanned model and establishing the geometrically independent tooth unit.

In the followings, an indirect bonding technique will be introduced and summarized based on a virtual setup from CAD/CAM transfer trays. For a more detailed discussion of this procedure, the reader can refer some publications (Fillion, 2007; 2010).

1.   Dental arch should be segmented into individual dental units perceived as geometric units (Fig. 16).
2.   Making the treatment plan, including extraction or non-extraction, stripping, final arch form. Such prescriptions are incorporated in 3Txer software®.
3.   After setup, according to the selected prescription, upper and lower arch are manually adjusted to fit the final treatment result. (Fig. 17 C, D).
4.   The virtual brackets are placed on the same horizontal plane and centered on each tooth. In this procedure, individual arch form (virtual arch) can be determined.(Fig. 17 E)
5.   Virtual transfer trays are constructed. A rapid-prototype machine constructs in real time the transfer tray (Fig. 18 A).
6.   Positioning the tray over the teeth and seating the tray (Fig. 18 B).

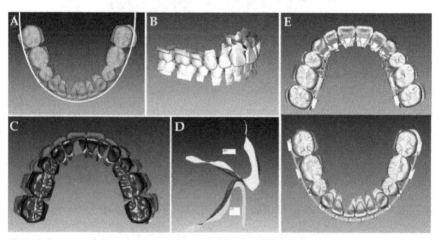

Fig. 17. **A**. Selection of the curve, on which the teeth will be positioned in construction of the set-up. **B**. Visualization of the set-up. **C, D**. Occlusion test: the red-colored zones represent the areas of contact. **E**. Precise positioning of the virtual brackets on the virtual set-up and placement of the ideal virtual arch wire.

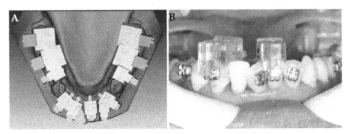

Fig. 18. **A**. Construction of the virtual transfer trays. **B**. Bonding of the brackets.

Material and equipment manufacturers continually introduce new and innovative products that further advance virtual technology. A fabrication procedure of virtual surgical splint procedure in virtual articulator has been also introduced, which spare the time consuming procedure of model surgery and surgical wafer fabrications (Song & Baek, 2009). Recently, a new imaging method, using computed tomography technology and laser scanning provides complete 3D views of the maxilla and the mandible, and the model setup with individual roots (Harrell *et al.*, 2002; Macchi *et al.*, 2006). The development of a 3D digital setup that displays individual crowns, roots and craniofacial structures will greatly help the clinician in diagnosis and treatment planning to determine various treatment options, monitor the changes after treatment over time, predict and display final treatment results, and measure treatment outcomes accurately (Macchi *et al.*, 2006).

Recently, Rangel and colleagues (Rangel *et al.*, 2008) reported the registration of digital models to 3D facial images. These multimodal images could improve our diagnosis and treatment planning processes and eventually will become the clinical standard, enhancing treatments provided by different specialties, including orthodontics, periodontics, prosthodontics, and restorative dentistry.

5. Introducing a novel method of the volumetric assessment of tooth wear using 3D reverse engineering technology

Tooth wear is defined as the non carious loss of tooth substance as a result of attrition, abrasion and erosion. Tooth attrition is regular and slow progressive loss of dental tissues as a consequence of tooth to tooth contact during mastication (Milicic *et al.*, 1987; Shafer *et al.*, 1983.) especially by parafunctions and unbalanced morphological occlusion.

Loss of occlusal surface of the tooth affects the vertical dimension and might induce deep bite (Ramjford & Ash, 1983). If there is attritional wear on the posterior teeth, they induce interference with completely seated TMJs and/or the anterior guidance (Dawson, 2007). High correlations among tooth wear, maximal bite force and the size of the gonial angle were reported (Kiliaridis *et al.*, 1995). Some previous studies reported the association between greater tooth wear and malocclusion (Carlsson *et al.*, 2003), although there were controversial opinions.

There are a few studies which investigated the relationship between tooth wear and orthodontic treatment (Kuijpers *et al.*, 2009). Until now there is no study focused on the tooth wear during orthodontic treatment, moreover no information about the quantity of tooth wear caused by orthodontic treatment. The main reason is probably due to the technical limit in quantifying the volumetric change of the tooth material. For that reason the most previous studies on tooth wear evaluated the tooth wear index only on study models. Recently, Cha *et al.* (Cha et al., 2007) suggested the clinical method of the quantifying volumetric change due to tooth wear by using 3D digital model superimposition.

The followings will show you how to use the superimposition method of 3D digital models to quantify the amount of central incisor wear occurred during the orthodontic treatment (Fig. 19).

The maxillary and mandibular dental casts were taken before and after orthodontic treatment and scanned by a laser surface scanning system (KOD300®, Orapix co. LTD, Seoul, Korea) with the reliability of 50 μm. 3D virtual models of central incisors were reconstructed and imported to a 3D reverse modeling software (Rapidform XOR3®, INUS Technology, Seoul, Korea) (Fig 19. A, B). The 3D images of central incisor before and after orthodontic treatment were superimposed with best-fitting method. As reference area, the middle third of labial and lingual surface of central incisor were used, because these areas are considered to be rarely affected by attritional wear and the pathologic condition of gingival(Fig. 19 C)

To calculate the volume of central incisor, the 3 boundary planes were constructed on the 3D images of central incisor before treatment (Fig. 19 D, E). We compared the volume of the central incisors before and after treatment in relation with the boundary planes and we arrived at the conclusion that the second one was smaller (Fig. 19 F, G).

This technology can be applied into a quite diverse area in dentistry, e.g. quantity evaluation of teeth after prosthetic or conservative treatments.

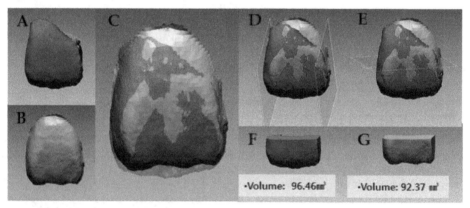

Fig. 19. Procedure for quantifying the amount of tooth wear. A. 3D digital model of maxillary incisor before orthodontic treatment (red). B. 3D digital model of the same tooth after orthodontic treatment (blue). C. Superimposition of A and B with best-fitting method using the middle third of labial and lingual surface as reference area. D, E. Mesial plane, distal plane, and gingival plane as boundary planes. F, G. 3D digital model before and after orthodontic treatment with the same boundary planes for volumetric calculation of tooth wear. The volume of tooth materials was reduced to about 4.09 mm³.

6. Presenting a quantitative 3D soft tissue facial analysis using a color coding system

Orthodontists have recognized that objective evaluation of facial morphology is important for the effective treatment planning and evaluation in reference to the growth change.

Traditionally, orthodontists have used radiographs to assess the soft tissue facial change, e.g. they measure 2D landmarks on the lateral cephalogram that arguably do not exist in a 3D body (Kau & Richmond, 2008). The problems in traditional cephalometrics also come from landmark identification of hard and soft tissues on x-rays because of the superimposition of several structures, which might be the major source of cephalometric errors. In the patient Fig. 20, it is showed that the facial contour angle was improved after orthognathic surgery but there is a limitation and difficulty to evaluate it at full extent three dimensionally.

Medical CT or Cone-beam CT (CBCT) can be an alternative, but possible overuse might lead to radiation exposure problems, together with financial burden. For the reason mentioned above, it should be stated that traditional longitudinal growth studies with radiation sources might present ethical and moral dilemmas. How to solve such an ethical dilemma? We think that the use of alternative surface imaging devices can be one step forward in handling such ethical dilemmas.

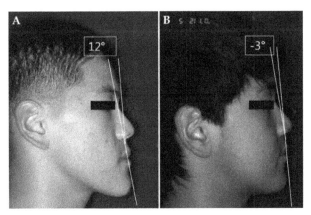

Fig. 20. **A**. Pre-treatment lateral view. **B**. Post-treatment lateral view. Note that although facial contour angle improved after surgery, there is a limitation to evaluate it at full extent.

With the advances in the technology, various devices, including laser scanners (Baik *et al.*, 2007), stereophotogrammetry (Ayoub *et al.*, 2003), and structured light systems (Weinberg *et al.*, 2004) have been used in acquiring the 3D images of the facial morphology. Among them, 3D laser scanner system or optical surface scanner is widely used because of its simple and rapid capture of the whole facial 3D image. It is quite likely that this system has a diverse possibility of clinical applications and researches (Baik *et al.*, 2007; Ismail & Moss, 2002; McCance *et al.*, 1997; McDonagh *et al.*, 2001; Moss, 2006; Moss *et al.*, 1995)

The laser scanning 3D technology allows to generate a high precision and can be used to calculate the morphological ground surface variations at different acquisition time intervals. The main advantages are that change due to growth or treatment of an individual can be monitored in three dimensions using this method, which is non-invasive and which can be repeated every few weeks (Moss, 2006; Moss *et al.*, 1995).

The registration program (Rapidform XOR3®, INUS technology, Seoul, Korea) enables superimposition of similar areas on two overlaid scans to demonstrate the surface differences in color coding system (Moss, 2006)(Fig. 22 E)

The purpose of 3D face registration is to align different 3D face data into a common coordinate system. So, registration is a crucial and indispensable step, as the accuracy of this step will greatly influence the performance of the whole face recognition system. The important step in the registration process is to determine which area will be used as a stable reference. The displacement, change in shape, or in size will be described relative to these structures. In the traditional 2D cephalometrics, the anterior cranial base e.g. Sella-Nasion is used for the superimpositions because of its relative stability after neural growth in brain. But locating 3D landmarks on complex curving structures is significantly more difficult (Miller et al., 2007; Morris et al., 1998; Moss et al., 1994).

Moss et al. (Moss *et al.*, 1994) combined five aforementioned anatomical landmarks (right and left endocanthion, right and left exocanthion and soft tissue Nasion) together with five constructed points projected onto the forehead. Hajeer et al. (Hajeer *et al.*, 2002) used seven superimposition points in the eye and nose area. Miller *et al.* (Miller et al., 2007) hold a view that the forehead area is stable area for superimposing 3D images. The superimposition points above were proved to be easy to locate and the landmarks well definable (Hoefert et al., 2010) (Fig. 21, Table 1).

There are, however, a number of problems that remain to be explored.

The forehead area with superimposition points 5, 6 and 7 in Fig. 21 and Table 1 were in an area, in which, according to the Bolton standards, 0.5 - 1.0 mm increase in Nasion-Sella line and a forward displacement of the frontal bone can be expected with normal growth in children between ages 4 and 5 (Hoefert et al., 2010). It means that the distance from sella turcica to foramen caecum does not increase after eruption of the first permanent molar and forehead can be used as a superimposing area.

However, this assumption is not supported by the mention that there was a correlation between frontal sinus pneumatization and the progression of skeletal maturity (Ruf & Pancherz, 1996). Another recent case reports by author (Cha *et al.*, 2011) provides the evidence that infraorbitale can be moved forward by maxillary protraction by using the surgical miniplate anchorage. These observations suggest further questions that must be reserved for a more extensive study.

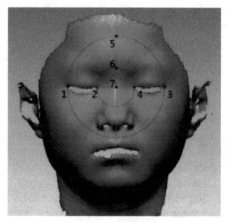

Fig. 21. Superimposition points (for explanation see Table 1).

Superimposition points	Description
Point 1	Right exocanthion
Point 2	Right endocanthion
Point 3	Left exocanthion
Point 4	Left endocanthion
Point 5	Intersection of forehead axis with the outer eye circle
Point 6	Intersection of forehead axis with the inner eye circle
Point 7	Middle of eye axis

Table 1. Superimposition points recommended by Hoefert *et al.* (Hoefert *et al.*, 2010).

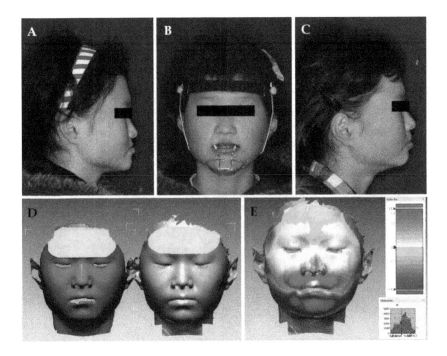

Fig. 22. 3D facial superimposition of the patient treated by maxillary protraction **A.** pre-treatment facial photo. **B.** Treatment by protraction headgear. **C.** Post-treatment facial photo. **D,E.** Superimposition of pre- and post-treatment 3D facial images using the forehead as reference area. According to the color-coding system, yellow/red color means forward movement, while blue color means backward movement.

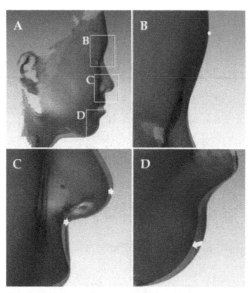

Fig. 23. **A.** Detailed sectional view of superimposition image in Fig. 22. **B.** Glabella was not changed. **C.** Nose tip and Subnasale was protruded by 0.6 mm and 1.2 mm, respectively. **D.** Pogonion was retruded in backward and downward direction by 2 mm.

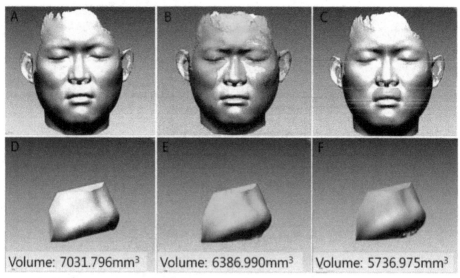

Fig. 24. Method for evaluating the volumetic change of the lip. **A~C.** 3D facial images were acquired and superimposition on forehead area was performed. To measure the volumetric change of the lip, boundary planes for the upper lip were constructed on the 3D facial images. **D~F.** The changes of lip volume before debonding (yellow), after debondig (green), and 6 months after debonding (blue).

Following is the example of the application of 3D facial registration for the evaluation of the change of facial morphology after orthopedic treatment. A patient who has a developing Class III malocclusion was monitored in order to assess the direction of growth and the rate of change after maxillary protraction therapy (Fig. 22 and 23).

There were no apparent changes to the central portion of the forehead and Glabella area (Fig. 23 B). There was general thickening of the lateral brow region, from 0.34 to 0.50 mm. The nose showed the positive change by 1.20 mm during the treatment (Fig. 23 C). There were visible but small positive changes in the cheek areas similar on both sides of the face. There was large and distinct forward and downward translation of the maxilla away from the forehead. There was elongation of the face leading to the downward projection of the soft-tissue chin (Fig. 23 D).

Another example (Fig. 24) represents the procedures for the evaluation of the quantitative change of lip volume between the final stage of the orthodontic treatment and after debonding procedure, to investigate the influence of bracket thickness for facial profile in 29 year-old male patients. The 3D facial images were imported into the Rapidform XOR3 software® (INUS technology, Seoul, Korea) and the superimposition method known as the best-fit was used on the reference area at the forehead, soft tissue glabella, including zygoma and nose.

To evaluate the volumetric change of the lip, 5 boundary planes were constructed on the 3D facial images. The volume in upper lip decreased 644.80 mm^3 immediately after debonding, and 650.01mm^3 more for the 6 month of retention period. The techniqueof the detailed volumetic measurement of soft tissue points to several promising applications for future research.

7. Presenting feasible methods of the integrating digital 3D model into a 3D facial image to visualize the anatomic position of the dentition

One area of high interest is the study of the integration of 3D digital model into a 3D facial image, which can be used as possible alternatives to 2D cephalometric superimposition. The 3D digital models of each dental arch are scanned independently and need to be related in space to represent the patient occlusion. Different methods have been developed for this purpose: visually assessing the study models' occlusion and matching their relative position in the virtual space; by scanning a wax bite, and registering the upper model to the upper side of the wax bite and the lower model to its lower side; by mounting the models in a bracket of known relative position, or by scanning the study models in occlusion and using that relative positional information to register the upper model to the lower one.

Rangel et al. (Rangel *et al.*, 2008) first introduced the procedure for the integration of 3D digital model in 3D facial image. Fig. 26 shows summarized procedures of digital model integration method.

For matching the 3D digital model to the 3D facial image, the anterior teeth were used as the registration surface.

1. To see the teeth on the 3D facial image, cheek retractors were used to pull the lips open, then a 3D facial image was made (Fig. 25 A and B).

2. A second 3D facial image was made from the patient at rest with the teeth in occlusion (Fig. 25 C).

3. 3D digital model is matched to the 3D facial image with the cheek retractors. To improve the accuracy of the registration, two step registration procedure were needed (Fig. 26 A~C).

4. Two 3D facial image at rest and with retractor were matched. Here as above, two step registration procedure were needed (Fig. 26 D~F).
5. Final 3D data set could be established (Fig. 27).

It seems technically possible to make a data set of a patient's face with the dentition positioned into this 3D picture. This procedure points to several promising applications for feature research about noncephalometric analysis or superimpositions.

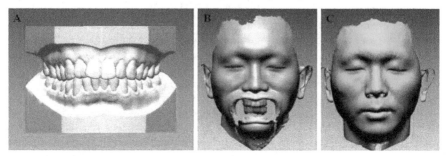

Fig. 25. **A.** 3D digital model. **B.** 3D facial image of the patient with cheek retractor. **C.** 3D facial image of the patient at rest position.

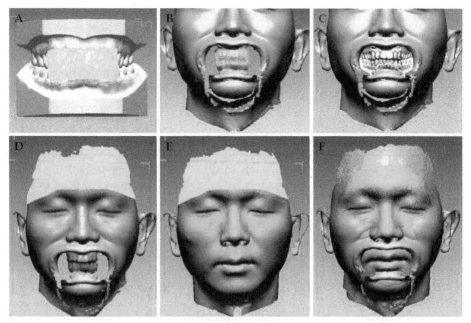

Fig. 26. Integration procedure of the 3D digital model into the 3D facial image. **A.** Region for surface registration is indicated on the 3D digital model(upper and lower anterior teeth were used). **B.** The same region in **A** is indicated on the 3D facial image with cheek retractor. **C.** Integration of 3D digital model and 3D facial image by using the registration area. **D, E.** Region for surface registration of two 3D facial images(forehead area was used). **F.** Superimposition of 3D facial images in **D** and **E**.

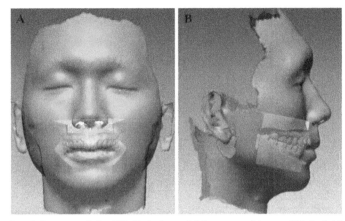

Fig. 27. Completed data set of the 3D digital model integrated into a 3D facial image. **A.** frontal view. **B.** profile view

8. Conclusion

In this chapter, we have reviewed the extent and limitation of the clinical application of 3D digital model and 3D facial image. The best-fit mathematical superimposition method of maxillary casts on the identical palatal vault is very accurate and allows for 3D evaluation of tooth movement. This technology can be also applied into a quite diverse area in dentistry, e.g. quantity evaluation of tooth material after conservative treatments or tooth wearing. The rapid development of CAD/CAM technology and the advances in 3D imaging of the face enable not only the virtual setup of the teeth but the results of treatment to be viewed from any perspective and to analyze the changes that have occurred by the treatment or growth.

9. References

Alcan, T.; Ceylanoglu, C. & Baysal, B. (2009). The relationship between digital model accuracy and time-dependent deformation of alginate impressions. *Angle Orthod*, Vol.79, No.1, pp. 30-36. ISSN 0003-3219

Ayoub, A.; Garrahy, A.; Hood, C.; White, J.; Bock, M.; Siebert, J.P.; Spencer, R. & Ray, A. (2003). Validation of a vision-based, three-dimensional facial imaging system. *Cleft Palate Craniofac J*, Vol.40, No.5, pp. 523-529. ISSN 1055-6656

Baik, H.S.; Jeon, J.M. & Lee, H.J. (2007). Facial soft-tissue analysis of Korean adults with normal occlusion using a 3-dimensional laser scanner. *Am J Orthod Dentofacial Orthop*, Vol.131, No.6, pp. 759-766. ISSN 1097-6752

Carlsson, G.E.; Egermark, I. & Magnusson, T. (2003). Predictors of bruxism, other oral parafunctions, and tooth wear over a 20-year follow-up period. *J Orofac Pain*, Vol.17, No.1, pp. 50-57. ISSN 1064-6655

Cha, B.K.; Choi, D.S.; Ngan, P.; Jost-Brinkmann, P.G.; Kim, S.M. & Jang, I.S. (2011). Maxillary protraction with miniplates providing skeletal anchorage in a growing Class III patient. *Am J Orthod Dentofacial Orthop*, Vol.139, No.1, pp. 99-112. ISSN 1097-6752

Cha, B.K.; Choi, J.I.; Jost-Brinkmann, P.G. & Jeong, Y.M. (2007). Applications of three-dimensionally scanned models in orthodontics. *Int J Comput Dent*, Vol.10, No.1, pp. 41-52. ISSN 1463-4201

Cha, B.K.; Lee, J.Y.; Jost-Brinkmann, P.G. & Yoshida, N. (2007). Analysis of tooth movement in extraction cases using three-dimensional reverse engineering technology. *Eur J Orthod*, Vol.29, No.4, pp. 325-331. ISSN 0141-5387

Choi, D.S.; Jeong, Y.M.; Jang, I.; Jost-Brinkmann, P.G. & Cha, B.K. (2010). Accuracy and reliability of palatal superimposition of three-dimensional digital models. *Angle Orthod*, Vol.80, No.4, pp. 497-503. ISSN 1945-7103

Costalos, P.A.; Sarraf, K.; Cangialosi, T.J. & Efstratiadis, S. (2005). Evaluation of the accuracy of digital model analysis for the American Board of Orthodontics objective grading system for dental casts. *Am J Orthod Dentofacial Orthop*, Vol.128, No.5, pp. 624-629. ISSN 0889-5406

Dalstra, M. & Melsen, B. (2009). From alginate impressions to digital virtual models: accuracy and reproducibility. *J Orthod*, Vol.36, No.1, pp. 36-41; discussion 14. ISSN 1465-3133

Dawson, P.E. (2007). *Functional occlusion: from TMJ to smile design*. Mosby. ISBN 978-0323033718, Philadelphia, USA

Eraso, F.E.; Parks, E.T.; Roberts, W.E.; Hohlt, W.F. & Ofner, S. (2007). Density value means in the evaluation of external apical root resorption: an in vitro study for early detection in orthodontic case simulations. *Dentomaxillofac Radiol*, Vol.36, No.3, pp. 130-137. ISSN 0250-832X

Fillion (2007). Computerized generated conception and fabrication of transfer trays for indirect bonding of lingual attachements: The Orapix system. *Rev Orthop Dento Facial*, Vol.41:1-15, pp. 1-15.

Ghafari, J.; Baumrind, S. & Efstratiadis, S.S. (1998). Misinterpreting growth and treatment outcome from serial cephalographs. *Clin Orthod Res*, Vol.1, No.2, pp. 102-106. ISSN 1397-5927

Gracco, A.; Buranello, M.; Cozzani, M. & Siciliani, G. (2007). Digital and plaster models: a comparison of measurements and times. *Prog Orthod*, Vol.8, No.2, pp. 252-259. ISSN 1723-7785

Hajeer, M.Y.; Ayoub, A.F.; Millett, D.T.; Bock, M. & Siebert, J.P. (2002). Three-dimensional imaging in orthognathic surgery: the clinical application of a new method. *Int J Adult Orthodon Orthognath Surg*, Vol.17, No.4, pp. 318-330. ISSN 0742-1931

Harrell, W.E., Jr.; Hatcher, D.C. & Bolt, R.L. (2002). In search of anatomic truth: 3-dimensional digital modeling and the future of orthodontics. *Am J Orthod Dentofacial Orthop*, Vol.122, No.3, pp. 325-330. ISSN 0889-5406

Hoefert, C.S.; Bacher, M.; Herberts, T.; Krimmel, M.; Reinert, S.; Hoefert, S. & Goz, G. (2010). Implementing a superimposition and measurement model for 3D sagittal analysis of therapy-induced changes in facial soft tissue: a pilot study. *J Orofac Orthop*, Vol.71, No.3, pp. 221-234. ISSN 1615-6714

Hoffman (1988). Indirect bonding with a diagnostic set-up. *J Clin Orthod*, Vol.8, pp. ISSN 509-511.

Horton, H.M.; Miller, J.R.; Gaillard, P.R. & Larson, B.E. (2009). Technique comparison for efficient orthodontic tooth measurements using digital models. *Angle Orthod*, Vol.80, No.2, pp. 254-261. ISSN 0003-3219

Ismail, S.F. & Moss, J.P. (2002). The three-dimensional effects of orthodontic treatment on the facial soft tissues--a preliminary study. *Br Dent J*, Vol.192, No.2, pp. 104-108. ISSN 0007-0610

Jang, I.; Tanaka, M.; Koga, Y.; Iijima, S.; Yozgatian, J.H.; Cha, B.K. & Yoshida, N. (2009). A novel method for the assessment of three-dimensional tooth movement during orthodontic treatment. *Angle Orthod*, Vol.79, No.3, pp. 447-453. ISSN 0003-3219

Kau, C.H. & Richmond, S. (2008). Three-dimensional analysis of facial morphology surface changes in untreated children from 12 to 14 years of age. *Am J Orthod Dentofacial Orthop*, Vol.134, No.6, pp. 751-760. ISSN 1097-6752

Keating, A.P.; Knox, J.; Bibb, R. & Zhurov, A.I. (2008). A comparison of plaster, digital and reconstructed study model accuracy. *J Orthod*, Vol.35, No.3, pp. 191-201; discussion 175. ISSN 1465-3125

Kiliaridis, S.; Johansson, A.; Haraldson, T.; Omar, R. & Carlsson, G.E. (1995). Craniofacial morphology, occlusal traits, and bite force in persons with advanced occlusal tooth wear. *Am J Orthod Dentofacial Orthop*, Vol.107, No.3, pp. 286-292. ISSN 0889-5406

Krejci, I.; Reich, T.; Bucher, W. & Lutz, F. (1994). [A new method for 3-dimensional wear measurement]. *Schweiz Monatsschr Zahnmed*, Vol.104, No.2, pp. 160-169. ISSN 1011-4203

Kuijpers, M.A.; Kiliaridis, S.; Renkema, A.; Bronkhorst, E.M. & Kuijpers-Jagtman, A.M. (2009). Anterior tooth wear and retention type until 5 years after orthodontic treatment. *Acta Odontol Scand*, Vol.67, No.3, pp. 176-181. ISSN 1502-3850 (Electronic)

Leifert, M.F.; Leifert, M.M.; Efstratiadis, S.S. & Cangialosi, T.J. (2009). Comparison of space analysis evaluations with digital models and plaster dental casts. *Am J Orthod Dentofacial Orthop*, Vol.136, No.1, pp. 16 e11-14; discussion 16. ISSN 1097-6752

Macchi, A.; Carrafiello, G.; Cacciafesta, V. & Norcini, A. (2006). Three-dimensional digital modeling and setup. *Am J Orthod Dentofacial Orthop*, Vol.129, No.5, pp. 605-610. ISSN 1097-6752

McCance, A.M.; Moss, J.P.; Fright, W.R.; Linney, A.D. & James, D.R. (1997). Three-dimensional analysis techniques--Part 2: Laser scanning: a quantitative three-dimensional soft-tissue analysis using a color-coding system. *Cleft Palate Craniofac J*, Vol.34, No.1, pp. 46-51. ISSN 1055-6656

McDonagh, S.; Moss, J.P.; Goodwin, P. & Lee, R.T. (2001). A prospective optical surface scanning and cephalometric assessment of the effect of functional appliances on the soft tissues. *Eur J Orthod*, Vol.23, No.2, pp. 115-126. ISSN 0141-5387

Milicic, A.; Gazi-Coklica, V. & Slaj, M. (1987). Dental attrition in preschool children. *Acta Stomatol Croat*, Vol.21, No.4, pp. 271-276. ISSN 0001-7019

Miller, L.; Morris, D.O. & Berry, E. (2007). Visualizing three-dimensional facial soft tissue changes following orthognathic surgery. *Eur J Orthod*, Vol.29, No.1, pp. 14-20. ISSN 0141-5387

Miller, R.J.; Kuo, E. & Choi, W. (2003). Validation of Align Technology's Treat III digital model superimposition tool and its case application. *Orthod Craniofac Res*, Vol.6 Suppl 1, pp. 143-149. ISSN 1601-6335

Morris, D.O.; Illing, H.M. & Lee, R.T. (1998). A prospective evaluation of Bass, Bionator and Twin Block appliances. Part II--The soft tissues. *Eur J Orthod*, Vol.20, No.6, pp. 663-684. ISSN 0141-5387

Moss, J.P. (2006). The use of three-dimensional imaging in orthodontics. *Eur J Orthod*, Vol.28, No.5, pp. 416-425. ISSN 0141-5387

Moss, J.P.; Linney, A.D. & Lowey, M.N. (1995). The use of three-dimensional techniques in facial esthetics. *Semin Orthod*, Vol.1, No.2, pp. 94-104. ISSN 1073-8746

Moss, J.P.; McCance, A.M.; Fright, W.R.; Linney, A.D. & James, D.R. (1994). A three-dimensional soft tissue analysis of fifteen patients with Class II, Division 1 malocclusions after bimaxillary surgery. *Am J Orthod Dentofacial Orthop*, Vol.105, No.5, pp. 430-437. ISSN 0889-5406

Myrberg, N.E. & Warner, C.F. (1982). Indirect bonding technique. *J Clin Orthod*, Vol.16, No.4, pp. 269-272. ISSN 0022-3875

Nagasaka, S.; Fujimura, T. & Segoshi, K. (2003). Development of a non-radiographic cephalometric system. *Eur J Orthod*, Vol.25, No.1, pp. 77-85. ISSN 0141-5387

Orapix (2010). *3Txer 3D virtual treatment planner*. Orapix www.orapix.com.

Ramjford, S.P. & Ash, M.M. (1983). *Occlusion*, W.B.Saunders, ISBN 978-0721655918, Philadelphia, USA

Rangel, F.A.; Maal, T.J.; Berge, S.J.; van Vlijmen, O.J.; Plooij, J.M.; Schutyser, F. & Kuijpers-Jagtman, A.M. (2008). Integration of digital dental casts in 3-dimensional facial photographs. *Am J Orthod Dentofacial Orthop*, Vol.134, No.6, pp. 820-826. ISSN 1097-6752

Ruf, S. & Pancherz, H. (1996). Frontal sinus development as an indicator for somatic maturity at puberty? *Am J Orthod Dentofacial Orthop*, Vol.110, No.5, pp. 476-482. ISSN 0889-5406

Santoro, M.; Galkin, S.; Teredesai, M.; Nicolay, O.F. & Cangialosi, T.J. (2003). Comparison of measurements made on digital and plaster models. *American journal of orthodontics and dentofacial orthopedics*, Vol.124, No.1, pp. 101-105. ISSN 0889-5406

Song, K.G. & Baek, S.H. (2009). Comparison of the accuracy of the three-dimensional virtual method and the conventional manual method for model surgery and intermediate wafer fabrication. *Oral Surg Oral Med Oral Pathol Oral Radiol Endod*, Vol.107, No.1, pp. 13-21. ISSN 1528-395X

Stevens, D.R.; Flores-Mir, C.; Nebbe, B.; Raboud, D.W.; Heo, G. & Major, P.W. (2006). Validity, reliability, and reproducibility of plaster vs digital study models: comparison of peer assessment rating and Bolton analysis and their constituent measurements. *American journal of orthodontics and dentofacial orthopedics*, Vol.129, No.6, pp. 794-803. ISSN 0889-5406

Weinberg, S.M.; Scott, N.M.; Neiswanger, K.; Brandon, C.A. & Marazita, M.L. (2004). Digital three-dimensional photogrammetry: evaluation of anthropometric precision and accuracy using a Genex 3D camera system. *Cleft Palate Craniofac J*, Vol.41, No.5, pp. 507-518. ISSN 1055-6656

Zachrisson, B.U. & Brobakken, B.O. (1978). Clinical comparison of direct versus indirect bonding with different bracket types and adhesives. *Am J Orthod*, Vol.74, No.1, pp. 62-78. ISSN 0002-9416

10

Recent Advances in the Genetics of Orthodontics

Yoko Tomoyasu, Tetsutaro Yamaguchi and Koutaro Maki
Department of Orthodontics, School of Dentistry, Showa University
Japan

1. Introduction

Consideration of genetic factors is an essential element of diagnosis that underlies orofacial traits. In particular, orthodontic clinicians may have an interest in craniofacial growth and tooth movement. These parts of the diagnostic process are important to understand the cause of the problem before attempting treatment. In this chapter, we present our studies on the genetic causes of external apical root resorption and mandibular morphology, and review related studies.

2. External apical root resorption (EARR)

External apical root resorption (EARR) is a common outcome following orthodontic treatment. The factors associated with this phenomenon are genetic background, the length of treatment, the magnitude of the orthodontic forces, the type of orthodontic movement, trauma and others (Brin & Bollen, 2011). Abnormal root shape is also a significant risk factor in root resorption (Kjaer, 1995). Allergy and asthma may also be high-risk factors for the development of excessive root resorption during orthodontic tooth movement (Nishioka et al., 2006).

Interleukin 1 beta IL-1B, a potent bone-resorptive cytokine, is a key component of the complex signaling pathways leading to root resorption. The proinflammatory cytokine IL-1 is a key mediator of the inflammatory response and regulates the proliferation of fibroblasts in the gingival and periodontal ligaments. The level of IL-1B notably increases in the human gingival crevicular fluid during orthodontic treatment (Uematsu et al., 1996). The levels of IL-1 correlate with individual differences in the amount of tooth translation (Iwasaki et al., 2001) and are thought to play a role in susceptibility to EARR (Davidovitch, 1991). Moreover, *IL-1B*-knockout mice demonstrate significantly greater root resorption than wild-type controls when undergoing experimental orthodontic treatments (Viecilli et al., 2009).

A C-to-T single nucleotide polymorphism (SNP) in *IL-1B*, rs1143634, may be causally associated with susceptibility to EARR. The TT genotype of this polymorphism has been associated with a 4-fold increase in IL-1B production (Pociot et al., 1992; di Giovine et al., 1995). Al-Qawasmi et al. (2003) reported an association of this polymorphism with the risk of EARR in the Caucasian population. Subjects homozygous for the C allele had a 5.6-fold

(95% confidence interval, 1.9–21.2) increased risk of EARR greater than 2 mm compared with those not homozygous for the C allele.

2.1 EARR and the Il-1B gene in the Japanese

Differences in tooth shape are used to characterize race and to provide an indication of racial affinity between human populations. For example, there are differences in the approximal root topography of teeth in the Chinese population compared with other populations (Ong & Neo, 1990). Sameshima & Sinclair (2001) reported that Asian patients experienced significantly less root resorption than Caucasian or Hispanic patients. We examined the association between a single polymorphism (rs1143634) in *IL-1B* and root resorption in 54 Japanese subjects (Tomoyasu et al., 2009a). Lateral cephalograms and panoramic radiographs were obtained from 54 Japanese subjects comprising 18 men and 36 women. The roots of three types of teeth were measured on pretreatment and posttreatment lateral cephalometric and panoramic radiographs. The roots of the maxillary and mandibular central incisors were measured from the pretreatment and posttreatment cephalometric radiographs. The mesial and distal roots of the left and right sides were measured on the panoramic radiographs. We amplified DNA by polymerase chain reaction, and genotyped the SNP by DNA sequencing. We found no significant difference between the genotype frequencies of the *IL-1B* SNP rs1143634 and the amount of root resorption in the Japanese population (Tables 1, 2).

	\multicolumn{4}{c}{Maxillary incisor (mm)}				\multicolumn{4}{c}{Mandibular incisor (mm)}			
	n	Mean	S.D.	P	n	Mean	S.D.	P
CC	45	2.1	2	0.29	48	1.7	1.5	0.86
CT	6	2.9	1.3		6	1.7	1.8	
	\multicolumn{4}{c}{Mandibular mesial incisor (mm)}				\multicolumn{4}{c}{Mandibular incisor (mm)}			
	n	Mean	S.D.	P	n	Mean	S.D.	P
CC	46	0.5	1.4	0.39	46	0.5	0.7	0.27
CT	6	0.7	1		6	1.2	1.6	

Table 1. The relationship between the *IL-1B* SNP rs1143634 and the amount of root resorption of the maxillary incisor, mandibular incisor, mandibular mesial molar, and mandibular distal molar in Japanese subjects. No statistical significance of the differences between the *IL-1B* genotype and the amount of root resorption was found.

	Unaffected groups (<2.0mm)		Affected groups (≥2.0mm)		
IL-1B marker	CC	CT	CC	CT	P
Maxillary central incisor	22	2	23	4	0.47
Mandibular central incisor	31	3	17	3	0.48
Mandibular first molar, mesial root	45	5	1	1	0.08
Mandibular first molar, distal root	44	5	2	1	0.22

Table 2. Relationship between the unaffected and affected groups by genotype. Subjects were classified as unaffected (<2.0 mm) or affected (≥2.0 mm), according to the amount of root resorption. No statistical significance of the differences between the *IL-1B* genotype and the classification of root resorption was determined.

2.2 Accuracy of EARR measurements

In our study, we failed to replicate in the Japanese population the previously reported association between the *IL-1B* polymorphism and EARR. In our study, we used lateral cephalograms to measure the amount of root resorption. In the study by Al-Qawasmi et al. (2003), lateral cephalograms and panoramic radiographs were used to measure EARR. However, the intraoral radiograph is more useful for measuring the amount of root resorption than the panoramic radiograph or lateral cephalogram. McFadden et al. (1989) indicated that errors in measurement using electronic calipers on lateral cephalometric films were approximately 2.5 times more frequent than the errors using periapical radiographs. Sameshima & Asgarifar (2001) suggested that the use of panoramic radiographs to measure root resorption might overestimate the amount of root loss by 20% or more, and that they are not as precise or reliable as intraoral radiographs (Bastos Lages et al., 2009).

To solve this problem, Bastos Lages et al. (2009) used periapical radiographs to determine the presence and severity of EARR to reduce the bias related to the diagnosis of EARR by other types of radiographs. In this report, the positive association was replicated in the Brazilian population.

They described that errors will certainly continue to occur until an accurate three-dimensional imaging system is available, because the accuracy of periapical x-rays for EARR measurements is unlikely that any inconsistencies in evaluating root resorption by this method in our study seriously biased the estimates of EARR.

2.3 Ethnic differences in the frequency of the *IL-1B* polymorphism

It is well known that differences in SNP frequencies among human populations are ethnicity-dependent (Wang et al., 2008). Ethnic factors are also considered to be a major variable in evaluating predisposition to EARR (Sameshima & Sinclair, 2001).

We characterized the ethnic variation at the *IL-1B* locus by examining the allele frequencies of the *IL-1B* polymorphism among individuals with different ethnic backgrounds. DNA samples from 24 Han Chinese, 24 African Americans, 24 European Americans, and 24 Hispanics were obtained, but no craniofacial measurements taken, and were used as reference populations for the allele frequencies of the *IL-1B* SNP.

There were marked differences in the frequency of the T allele of rs1143634 among the various ethnic populations (Table 3). The highest frequency (29.2%) was observed in the European Caucasians. The African American and Hispanic populations carried the T allele at frequencies of 10.4% and 14.7%, respectively. In contrast, the Japanese and Han Chinese populations carried the T allele at the markedly lower frequencies of 5.6% and 2.5%, respectively.

	Japanese	Han Chinese	African American	European Caucasian	Hispanic
n	54	24	24	24	24
C	94.4%	97.5%	89.6%	70.8%	85.3%
T	5.6%	2.5%	10.4%	29.2%	14.7%

Table 3. Allele distribution of the *IL-1B* SNP rs1143634 among different ethnicities.

The marked allelic diversity between different ethnic groups at this locus may explain our failure to identify any association between rs1143634 and EARR in the Japanese. We observed that Asian populations have a higher frequency of the C allele than other ethnic groups. In our data, only six Japanese subjects had a T allele. The failure to detect an association between the rs1143634 and root resorption in the Japanese may be due to the study being underpowered to detect a polymorphism that occurs at a relatively low frequency. In contrast, in the populations in which positive associations with EARR were identified, namely Caucasians and Brazilians, the T allele occurs at a higher frequency (Caucaisans: C; 70.8%, T; 29.2%, Tomoyasu et al., 2009a) (Brazilians: C; 43.4%, T; 56.6%, Bastos Lages et al., 2009), respectively. Further studies evaluating the genetic determinants of root resorption susceptibility are required.

3. Mandibular morphology and the growth hormone receptor gene

Craniofacial morphology has a strong genetic component but it is also influenced by environmental factors, making it a complex trait to study. Growth hormone (GH) is a craniofacial morphological determinant; it plays a major role in the growth and development of the craniofacial complex by directly and indirectly modulating the size and the angular relationships of the craniofacial structures (Ramirez-Yanez et al., 2005). Children with deficient or excess GH have been reported to develop unique craniofacial configurations (Pirinen et al., 1994). Disproportionate growth of the cranial base structures and jaws results in facial retrognathia, which entails a proportionately smaller posterior than anterior facial height in persons of short stature with GH deficiency (Kjelberg et al., 2000). GH therapy for children with short stature or Turner syndrome results in characteristic patterns of craniofacial growth (Van Erum et al., 1988; Simmons, 1999). Responses to systemic GH therapy are time- and site-dependent in the craniofacial region, and are associated with an increase in cartilage growth, particularly within the mandibular ramus (Van Erum et al., 1988; Simmons, 1999). Children who receive long-term GH replacement therapy show exaggerated growth of the craniofacial skeleton, especially with respect to the height of the mandibular ramus (Funatsu et al., 2006; Forsberg et al., 2002). A comparison of children with Turner syndrome who received recombinant human GH treatment and a large cross-sectional control group showed a statistically significant increase in ramus growth associated with mandibular ramus height, but not with mandibular body length, maxillary length, or anterior cranial base length (Rongen-Westerlaken et al., 1993).

Growth hormone receptors (GHRs) have been shown by molecular genetic analysis to be present in the mandibular condyle (Lewinson et al., 1994). Analysis of the *Ghr* knockout mouse has revealed that the GH→GHR→insulin-like growth factor 1 system is important in postnatal growth and that GHR plays a role in maintaining proportional skeletal growth (Sjogren et al., 2000). In *Ghr* knockout mice, the height of the mandibular ramus is significantly reduced (Ramirez-Yanez et al., 2005), and disproportionate skeletal growth is reflected by decreased femur:crown-rump and femur:tibia ratios (Sjogren et al., 2000). There are diverse mutations and polymorphisms in the *GHR* gene in humans. Reports have shown a relationship between *GHR* and idiopathic short stature (Goddard et al., 1995) and Laron syndrome (growth hormone insensitivity syndrome), which is marked by a characteristic facial appearance. Interestingly, patients with GHR deficiency showed significantly decreased vertical facial growth (Schaefer et al., 1994). Therefore, GHR is suggested to have site-, area-, or region-specific effects (Hartsfield, 2005).

3.1 Relationship between the *GHR* gene and mandibular morphology in the Japanese

We quantitatively evaluated the relationship between craniofacial morphology and the P561T variant in exon 10 of the *GHR* gene in the non-syndromic Japanese population (Yamaguchi et al., 2001). DNA and cephalograms were obtained from 50 Japanese men and 50 Japanese women. To analyze craniofacial morphology, measurements were made on tracings of lateral cephalograms under standardized conditions. We measured cranial base length (nasion–sella; N–S), maxillary length (point A-pterygomaxillary fissure; A'–PTM'), overall mandibular length (gnathion–condylion; Gn–Co), mandibular corpus length (pogonion–gonion; Pog'–Go), and mandibular ramus height (condylion–gonion; Co–Go) (Figure 1). Body height was also measured. We identified a significant association of the polymorphic GHR gene (P561T, rs6184) with mandibular ramus height ($P = 0.0181$) (Table 4).

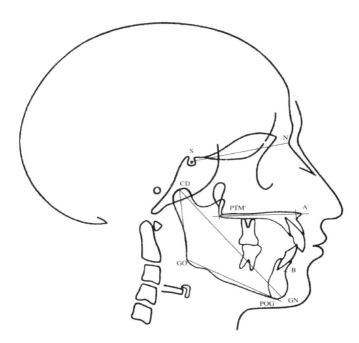

Fig. 1. Cephalometric reference points and lines used to assess the relationship between *GHR* gene variants. N–S, cranial base length; A'–PTM', maxillary length; Co–Go, mandibular ramus length; Pog'–Go; mandibular corpus length; Gn–Co, overall mandibular length.

	P561T	n	Body Height (cm)	N-S (mm)	A'-PTM' (mm)	Gn-Co (mm)
Subjects	CC	86	165.2±7.8	71.0±3.6	50.9±3.3	126.3±9.5
(100)	CA	14	163.4±10.5	70.0±4.6	50.4±3.7	122.3±9.6
	P		0.32	0.6	0.47	0.12
Men	CC	44	171.0±5.5	72.6±3.6	52.1±3.1	131.6±7.0
(50)	CA	6	173.7±6.5	72.6±5.1	53.0±3.5	131.4±7.4
	P		0.4	0.55	0.53	0.98
Women	CC	42	159.2±4.6	69.3±2.7	49.6±3.0	120.7±8.6
(50)	CA	8	155.6±3.9	68.1±3.3	48.4±2.5	115.5±3.1
	P		0.38	0.32	0.26	0.06

	P561T	n	Pog'-Go(mm)	Co-Go(mm)	Height/Co-Go
Subjects	CC	86	81.2±6.0	63.5±6.9	2.7±0.2
(100)	CA	14	79.3±7.2	58.9±6.1	2.9±0.3
	P		0.32	.018*	.013*
Men	CC	44	84.3±4.7	68.5±4.4	2.5±0.2
(50)	CA	6	86.3±3.7	64.9±2.1	2.7±0.1
	P		0.37	.021*	.015*
Women	CC	42	78.0±5.6	58.3±4.9	2.8±0.3
(50)	CA	8	74.2±3.7	54.4±3.5	2.9±0.3
	P		0.07	.025*	.028*

Table 4. The relationship between *GHR* gene variants and linear measurements in 50 men and 50 women. *P < 0.05.

To confirm these findings, we extended our previous study, genotyping approximately 1.7-times more non-syndromic Japanese individuals than analyzed in a previous report. Genomic DNA and lateral cephalograms were obtained from 167 Japanese subjects comprising 50 men and 117 women. The male subjects were the same as those we reported previously. We genotyped these individuals for five SNPs in the coding region of GHR (exon 10): C422F (rs6182, GG and GT genotype), S473S (rs6176, CC and CT genotype), P477T (rs6183, CC and CA genotype), I526L (rs6180, AA, AC and CC genotype), and P561T (rs6184, CC and CA genotype). We identified a significant relationship between the P56IT and C422F genotypes with mandibular ramus height in the Japanese population (P < 0.05; Table 5). These two polymorphisms are in linkage disequilibrium (Tomoyasu et al., 2009b).

		n	Body height (cm)			N-S (mm)		
			Mean	S.D.	P	Mean	S.D.	P
C422F	GG	135	161.6	7.9	0.16	69.7	3.4	0.66
	GT	16	164.6	10.2		69.3	4.4	
S473S	CC	137	161.9	8.4	0.95	69.6	3.5	0.32
	CT	11	161.1	6.1		70.5	2.8	
P477T	CC	146	161.6	8.3	0.47	69.6	3.5	0.58
	CA	4	163.8	9.1		69.5	4.8	
I526L	AA	77	162.7	8.8	0.47	69.5	3.5	0.56
	AC	44	161	7.9		70.2	4	
	CC	32	161.4	6.9		69.4	2.6	
P561T	CC	135	161.6	7.9	0.16	69.7	3.4	0.66
	CA	16	164.6	10.2		69.3	4.4	

		n	A'-PTM' (mm)			Gn-Co (mm)		
			Mean	S.D.	P	Mean	S.D.	P
C422F	GG	135	50	4.8	0.95	122.9	9.3	0.63
	GT	16	49.9	3.1		121.7	8.5	
S473S	CC	137	49.9	4.8	0.71	122.9	9.2	0.89
	CT	11	49.8	2.1		123	9.7	
P477T	CC	146	49.9	4.7	0.54	122.7	9.1	0.15
	CA	4	51.3	3.5		130.5	11.4	
I526L	AA	77	50.1	3.2	0.06	124.2	9.7	0.19
	AC	44	50.7	3.1		121.6	8.7	
	CC	32	48.1	7.9		121.4	7.7	
P561T	CC	135	50	4.8	0.95	122.9	9.3	0.63
	CA	16	49.9	3.1		121.7	8.5	

		n	Pog'-Go (mm)			Co-Go (mm)		
			Mean	S.D.	P	Mean	S.D.	P
C422F	GG	135	79.5	5.6	0.78	61.6	6.5	0.02*
	GT	16	79.9	7.2		57.9	6.1	
S473S	CC	137	79.9	5.9	0.31	61.5	6.5	0.54
	CT	11	78.5	6.4		60.9	5.6	
P477T	CC	146	79.8	6	0.23	61.3	6.4	0.17
	CA	4	83.3	5.7		65.6	4.5	
I526L	AA	77	80.1	5.8	0.82	62.4	6.7	0.13
	AC	44	79.6	5.5		61.1	6.8	
	CC	32	79.5	6.8		59.7	5.4	
P561T	CC	135	79.5	5.6	0.78	61.6	6.5	0.02*
	CA	16	79.9	7.2		57.9	6.1	

Table 5. Relationship between 5 SNPs in the GHR and 6 linear measurements of body height and craniofacial morphology in 167 Japanese subjects. *P < 0.05.

	n	Body height(cm)			N-S (mm)		
		Mean	S.D.	P	Mean	S.D.	P
d3/fl-GHR							
fl/fl	92	171.2	7.2	0.24	75.3	3.8	0.92
fl/d3	24	169.7	6.3		75.6	3.8	
d3/d3	9	173.7	3.9		75.4	4.4	
C422F/P561T							
GG/CC	124	170.6	7.1	0.49	75.2	3.8	0.7
GT/CA	24	169.6	6.7		75.2	3.7	
S473S							
CC	145						
CT	3						
P477T							
CC	145						
CA	3						
I526L							
AA	62	171.5	7.2	0.19	75.8	3.7	0.24
AC	61	170	7.2		74.8	3.3	
CC	24	169	6.3		75.1	4.5	

	n	A'-PTM'(mm)			Gn-Co (mm)		
		Mean	S.D.	P	Mean	S.D.	P
d3/fl-GHR							
fl/fl	92	52	3.2	0.79	139.6	8.3	0.21
fl/d3	24	52.2	3.4		137.8	6.9	
d3/d3	9	51.3	2.5		142.7	10.4	
C422F/P561T							
GG/CC	124	52.1	3.3	0.32	138.7	8	0.38
GT/CA	24	51.3	2.9		137.7	8.6	
S473S							
CC	145						
CT	3						
P477T							
CC	145						
CA	3						
I526L							
AA	62	52.6	3.2	0.24	139.1	8.7	0.71
AC	61	51.7	3.2		137.9	7.8	
CC	24	51.7	3.7		139.2	7.9	

	n	Pog'-Go(mm)			Co-Go(mm)		
		Mean	S.D.	P	Mean	S.D.	P
d3/fl-GHR							
fl/fl	92	84.8	5.5	0.12	72	7.6	0.59
fl/d3	24	82.8	5.2		70.7	6.3	
d3/d3	9	84.5	4.5		72.5	6.6	
C422F/P561T							
GG/CC	124	83.9	5.5	0.77	71.9	7.1	0.02*
GT/CA	24	84.2	5.3		68.5	5.5	
S473S							
CC	145						
CT	3						
P477T							
CC	145						
CA	3						
I526L							
AA	62	84.3	5.7	0.82	72	7.6	0.68
AC	61	83.5	5.3		71.2	6.5	
CC	24	84.2	84.2		71.1	7.4	

Table 6. The relationship between six SNPs in GHR and six linear measurements of body height and craniofacial morphology in 159 Korean subjects. *P < 0.05.

3.2 Relationship between the *GHR* gene and mandibular morphology in Asian populations

Following our report of an association between an exon 10 SNP in the *GHR* gene and mandibular ramus height in the Japanese (Yamaguchi et al., 2001), Zhou et al. (2005) reported the association of another exon 10 *GHR* polymorphism, I526L, with mandibular height in 95 Han Chinese subjects. We did not replicate this finding in 167 Japanese subjects (Tomoyasu et al., 2009b).

We also evaluated the association of *GHR* polymorphisms with mandibular ramus height in the Korean population (Kang et al., 2009). Genomic DNA samples and lateral cephalograms were obtained from 159 Korean subjects, comprising 100 men and 59 women. We tested the five aforementioned exon 10 SNPs plus a common polymorphism *d3/fl-GHR* that results in genomic deletion of exon 3 (Urbanek et al., 1992; Pantel et al., 2000). Two common isoforms of GHR, one full-length (fl-GHR) and the other lacking the extracellular domain encoded by exon 3 (d3-GHR), are associated with differences in responsiveness to GH. Children carrying at least one *d3-GHR* allele show a 1.7- to 2-fold greater response to GH than do *fl-GHR/fl-GHR* homozygotes (Dos-Santos et al., 2004). This common polymorphism has also been associated with the degree of height increase in response to GH therapy in French children of short stature who were born small for gestational age or with idiopathic short stature (Dos-Santos et al., 2004), as well as in German Turner syndrome patients (Binder et al., 2006), and Brazilian GH-deficient children (Jorge et al., 2006).

Table 6 shows the frequencies of the six *GHR* genotypes and the relationships between these genotypes and six linear measurements of body height and craniofacial morphology in 159 Korean subjects. Heterozygosity for S473S and P477T (genotypes CT and CA, respectively) was found in only three subjects. Therefore, statistical analysis was not performed for S473S or P477T. Genotype-specific association analysis revealed that mandibular ramus height only was significantly correlated with the P561T (a C-to-A transversion) and C422F (a G-to-T transversion) variants ($P = 0.024$). The *d3/fl-GHR* polymorphism was not associated with any measurement. These data replicated our findings in the Japanese population, but were different from the findings reported for the Han Chinese population.

We confirmed an association between polymorphisms P561T and C422F and mandibular ramus height. Individuals with the genotype CC for polymorphism P561T and the genotype GG for polymorphism C422F had a significantly greater mandibular height than those with genotypes CA and GT, respectively.

3.3 Ethnic differences in the *GHR* SNP allele frequencies

A clue to understanding ethnic differences in the association between the *GHR* locus and mandibular ramus height might be gained by determining the allelic frequencies of the five SNPs among 24 Han Chinese, 24 African Americans, 24 European Americans, and 24 Hispanics. we examined the allelic frequencies of the five SNPs among 24 Han Chinese, 24 African Americans, 24 European Americans, and 24 Hispanics. We found that the allele frequencies vary considerably (Table 7).

The reason for the difference between Japanese/Koreans and Chinese remains unclear; however, we did find widely discordant allele frequencies in the *GHR* exon 10 SNPs between some of the different ethnic groups. Indeed, the association of *GHR* is different depending on ethnicity in other cases, such as Laron syndrome (Hopp et al., 1996; Shevah et al., 2004) and idiopathic short stature (Blum et al., 2006; Hujeirat et al., 2006; Bonioli et al.,

2005; Sjoberg et al., 2001; Sanchez et al., 1998; Johnston et al., 2000). These differences might imply the need for independent studies on the association of *GHR* with craniofacial morphology in each ethnic group. The mandibular size of Japanese people appears to be slightly smaller than that of European-Americans (Miyajima et al., 1996) or Caucasians (Ishii et al., 2001; Ishii et al., 2002; Ishizuka et al., 1989).

		Japanese (n=167)	Han Chinese (n=24)	African American (n=24)	European American (n=24)	Hispanic (n=24)
C422F	G	94.1%	79.4%	100.0%	100.0%	100.0%
	T	5.9%	20.6%	0.0%	0.0%	0.0%
S473S	C	96.3%	97.3%	100.0%	97.5%	100.0%
	T	3.7%	2.6%	0.0%	2.5%	0.0%
P477T	C	98.7%	100.0%	100.0%	100.0%	100.0%
	A	1.3%	0.0%	0.0%	0.0%	0.0%
I526L	A	46.7%	38.2%	64.3%	58.3%	62.4%
	C	53.3%	61.8%	35.6%	41.6%	37.5%
P561T	C	94.7%	80.0%	100.0%	100.0%	100.0%
	A	5.2%	19.9%	0.0%	0.0%	0.0%

Table 7. Allele distribution of 5 SNPs in exon10 of the GHR

On average, the allele frequencies for populations from different continents differ by 16–19%, and for populations within a continent, such as Koreans and Japanese, they differ by 5–10% (Miller et al., 2005). These differences may be sufficiently large, even among the closely related Korean, Japanese, and Chinese populations, to cause substructural problems for case–control genetic studies of complex traits. Indeed, our findings in the Japanese and Korean populations were not replicated in the Han Chinese. A haplotype-based study based on HapMap data is required to assess the differences among Asian populations, and a larger-scale study with the ethnicities kept distinct is required to obtain a conclusive result (Roeder et al., 2006; Ambrosius et al., 2004; Schork et al., 2002; Longmate et al., 2001). Our work emphasizes the importance of close matching of ethnic groups, especially when measuring craniofacial morphology, which is known to vary by ethnicity (Miyajima et al., 1996; Ishii et al., 2001; Ishii et al., 2002; Ioi et al., 2007).

Growth hormone insensitivity syndrome of genetic origin has been linked to many different mutations of *GHR*, and is associated with a wide range of severities of clinical and biochemical phenotypes. Mandibular growth is also influenced by multiple factors, among which heterozygous *GHR* mutations appear to play a more or less important role, depending on the kind of mutation and on the overall genetic make-up of the individual. Although there is continuing interest in the functional importance of the P56IT and C422F variants, their precise roles remain unknown. The availability of an environmental factor (*i.e.*, orthopedic treatment) has made it possible to initiate therapeutic trials on children with short ramus height. Sasaki et al. (2007) reported a Japanese patient with ectodermal dysplasia, and proposed that the P561T variant could be a genetic marker for mandibular growth. Sasaki et al. (2009) reported that a difference in mandibular growth between P561T heterozygous and wild-type individuals could be demonstrated by cephalometric measurements during childhood. A heterozygous P561T mutation may affect mandibular growth during early childhood, as it is hypothesized to function as an inhibitory factor in the process of mandibular growth. *GHR* is considered a possible genetic marker for mandibular ramus height (Sasaki et al., 2007). This genetic factor might be considered along with other factors associated with mandibular growth when planning treatment to influence mandibular height, such as Herbst appliances, functional appliances, headgear, and facemask therapy.

3.4 Mandibular prognathism

We previously reported a genome-wide linkage analysis with 90 mandibular prognathism sib-pairs from an Asian population, and identified three significantly linked chromosomal loci: 1p36, 6q25, and 19p13.2 (Yamaguchi et al., 2005). These do not include the *GHR* locus on chromosome 5. We did not find any *GHR* gene SNPs that were associated with mandibular corpus length or overall mandibular length; there was also no identified association in the Chinese population (Zhou et al., 2005).

Recently, there have been four reports describing mandibular prognathism-related genes or loci. Jang et al. (2010) reported that polymorphisms in matrilin-1 could be used as a marker for genetic susceptibility to mandibular prognathism. Xue et al. (2010) reported an association between genetic polymorphisms in the erythrocyte membrane protein band 4.1 gene and mandibular prognathism. Li et al. (2010, 2011) reported a novel suggestive linkage locus for mandibular prognathism in two Chinese pedigrees. The linked region, around SNP rs875864 on chromosome 4, contains candidate genes include *EVC* and *EVC2* (Li et al., 2010), and that on chromosome 4 between rs1468507 and rs7141857 contains candidate genes including transforming growth factor, beta 3 and latent transforming growth factor beta binding protein (Li et al., 2011). Further studies will be needed to find the rare variants causing mandibular prognathism.

3.5 Conclusion

While various environmental factors contribute to morphogenesis of the mandible, genetic factors play a substantial role (Chang et al., 2006). However, there are very few reports that have examined the correlation between craniofacial morphology and genotype. Our studies have succeeded in elucidating susceptibility locus-related non-syndromic craniofacial morphology. We have also found marked diversities in the allelic frequencies of GH receptor polymorphisms within a multi-ethnic study population, which might partly explain the differing craniofacial morphologies among different ethnicities. Recent advances in clinical genetics have increased our knowledge of the genetic impact on craniofacial phenotypes. Identifying the genetic susceptibility for specific craniofacial phenotypes would enable more effective diagnosis and treatment for patients while they were still growing.

4. Acknowledgments

We are deeply grateful to the study participants. We also thank our collaborators, Ituro Inoue (National Institute of Genetics), Atsushi Tajima (Tokushima University), Ryosuke Kimura (University of the Ryukyus), Soo Byung Park (Pusan National University), Miyuki Watanabe (Showa University), Masaaki Yamaguchi (Showa University), and Yoshinobu Shibasaki (Showa University). The protocols used in our studies were approved by the relevant Ethics Committees, and all patients gave their written informed consent to participate in the study before samples were taken. The dbSNP numbers are taken from the dbSNP database at the National Center for Biotechnology Information. (http://www.ncbi.nlm.nih.gov/SNP/)

5. References

Al-Qawasmi, RA.; Hartsfield, JK Jr.; Everett, ET.; Flury, L.; Liu, L.; Foroud, TM. et al. (2003). Genetic predisposition to external apical root resorption. *Am J Orthod Dentofacial Orthop*, Vol. 123, No. 3, pp. 242-252, ISSN 0889-5406

Ambrosius, WT.; Lange, EM. & Langefeld, CD. (2004). Power for genetic association studies with random allele frequencies and genotype distributions. *Am J Hum Genet*, Vol. 74, No. 4, pp. 683-693, ISSN 0002-9297

Bastos Lages, EM.; Drummond, AF.; Pretti, H.; Costa, FO.; Lages, EJ.; Gontijo, AI. et al. (2009). Association of functional gene polymorphism IL-1beta in patients with external apical root resorption. *Am J Orthod Dentofacial Orthop*, Vol. 136, No. 4, pp. 542-546, ISSN 1097-6752

Binder, G.; Baur, F.; Schweizer, R. & Ranke, MB. (2006). The d3-growth hormone receptor polymorphism is associated with increased responsiveness to GH in Turner syndrome and short SGA children. *J Clin Endocrinol Metab*, Vol. 91, No. 2, pp. 659–664, ISSN 0021-972X

Blum, WF.; Machinis, K.; Shavrikova, EP.; Keller, A.; Stobbe, H.; Pfaeffle, RW. et al. (2006). The growth response to growth hormone (GH) treatment in children with isolated GH deficiency is independent of the presence of the exon 3-minus isoform of the GH receptor. J Clin Endocrinol Metab, Vol. 91, No. 10, pp. 4171-4174, ISSN 0021-972X

Bonioli, E.; Taro, M.; Rosa, CL.; Citana, A.; Bertorelli, R.; Morcaldi, G. et al. (2005). Heterozygous mutations of growth hormone receptor gene in children with idiopathic short stature. *Growth Horm IGF Res*, Vol. 15, No. 6, pp. 405-410, ISSN 1096-6374

Brin, I.; Bollen, AM. (2011). External apical root resorption in patients treated by serial extractions followed by mechanotherapy. *Am J Orthod Dentofacial Orthop*, Vol. 139, No. 2, pp. e129-134, ISSN 1097-6752

Chang, HP.; Tseng, YC. & Chang, HF. (2006). Treatment of mandibular prognathism. *J Formos Med Assoc*, Vol. 105, No. 10, pp. 781-790, ISSN 0929-6646

Davidovitch Z. (1991). Tooth movement. *Crit Rev Bio Med*, Vol. 2, No. 4, pp. 411-450, ISSN 1045-4411

di Giovine, FS.; Cork, MJ.; Crane, A.; Mee, JB. & Duff, GW. (1995). Novel genetic association of an IL-1B gene variation a +3953 with IL-1B protein production and psoriasis. *Cytokine*, Vol. 7, No. 6, pp. 606, ISSN 1043-4666

Dos-Santos, C.; Essioux, L.; Teinturier, C.; Tauber, M.; Goffin, V. & Bougneres, P. (2004). A common polymorphism of the growth hormone receptor is associated with increased responsiveness to growth hormone. *Nat Genet*, Vol. 36, No. 7, pp. 720-724, ISSN 1061-4036

Forsberg, CM.; Krekmanova, L. & Dahllof, G. (2002). The effect of growth hormone therapy on mandibular and cranial base development in children treated with total body irradiation. *Eur J Orthod*, Vol. 24, No. 3, pp. 285–292, ISSN 0141-5387

Funatsu, M.; Sato, K. & Mitani, H. (2006). Effects of growth hormone on craniofacial growth. *Angle Orthod*, Vol. 76, No. 6, pp. 970–977, ISSN 0003-3219

Goddard, AD.; Covello, R.; Luoh, SM.; Clackson, T.; Attie, KM.; Gesundheit, N. et al. (1995). Mutations of the growth hormone receptor in children with idiopathic short stature. The Growth Hormone Insensitivity Study Group. *N Engl J Med*, Vol. 333, No. 17, pp. 1093-1098, ISSN 0028-4793

Hartsfield, JK. (2005). Genetics and Orthodontics, In: *Orthodontics: Current Principles & Techniques, 4th ed.*, Graber, TM.; Vanarsdall, RL. & Vig, KWL, pp. 101-115, Mosey, ISBN 0323026214, St. Louis

Hopp, M.; Rosenbloom, AL.; Griffiths, J.; Kgwete, S. & Vaccarello, MA. (1996). Growth hormone receptor deficiency (Laron syndrome) in black African siblings. *S Afr Med J*, Vol. 86, No. 3, pp. 268-270, ISSN 0256-9574

Hujeirat, Y.; Hess, O.; Shalev, S. & Tenenbaum-Rakover, Y. (2006). Growth hormone receptor sequence changes do not play a role in determining height in children with idiopathic short stature. *Horm Res*, Vol. 65, No. 4, pp. 210-216, ISSN 0301-0163

Ioi, H.; Nakata, S.; Nakasima, A. & Counts, AL. (2007). Comparison of cephalometric norms between Japanese and Caucasian adults in anteroom-posterior and vertical dimension. *Eur J Orthod*, Vol. 29, No. 5, pp. 493–499, ISSN 0141-5387

Ishii, N.; Deguchi, T. & Hunt, NP. (2001). Craniofacial morphology of Japanese girls with Class II division 1 malocclusion. *J Orthod*, Vol. 28, No. 3, pp. 211-215, ISSN 1465-3125

Ishii, N.; Deguchi, T. & Hunt, NP. (2002). Morphological differences in the craniofacial structure between Japanese and Caucasian girls with Class II Division 1 malocclusions. *Eur J Orthod*, Vol. 24, No. 1, pp. 61-67, ISSN 0141-5387

Ishizuka, K.; Yamazaki, T.; Inoue, K.; Kouchi, K.; Ou, B. & Namura, S. (1989). A morphological study of the cranial base and dentofacial structure of Japanese with Angle Class II, div. 1 malocclusion--as compared with American white with Angle Class II, div. 1 malocclusion. *Nippon Kyosei Shika Gakkai Zasshi*, Vol. 48, No. 1, pp. 1-6, ISSN 0021-454X

Iwasaki, LR.; Haack, JE.; Nickel, JC.; Reinhardt, RA. & Petro, TM. (2001). Human interleukin-1 beta and interleukin-1 receptor antagonist secretion and velocity of tooth movement. *Arch Oral Biol*, Vol. 46, No. 2, pp. 185-189, ISSN 0003-9969

Jang, JY.; Park, EK.; Ryoo, HM.; Shin, HI.; Kim, TH.; Jang, JS. et al. (2010). Polymorphisms in the Matrilin-1 gene and risk of mandibular prognathism in Koreans. *J Dent Res*, Vol. 89, No. 11, pp. 1203-1207, ISSN 1544-0591

Johnston, LB.; Pashankar, F.; Camacho-Hubner, C.; Savage, MO. & Clark, AJ. (2000). Analysis of the intracellular signalling domain of the human growth hormone receptor in children with idiopathic short stature. *Clin Endocrinol*, Vol. 52, No. 4, pp. 463-469, ISSN 0300-0664

Jorge, AA.; Marchisotti, FG.; Montenegro, LR.; Carvalho, LR.; Mendonca, BB. & Arnhold, IJ. (2006). Growth hormone (GH) pharmacogenetics: influence of GH receptor exon 3 retention or deletion on first-year growth response and final height in patients with severe GH deficiency. *J Clin Endocrinol Metab*, Vol. 91, No. 2, pp. 1076–1080, ISSN 0021-972X

Kang, EH.; Yamaguchi, T.; Tajima, A.; Nakajima, T.; Tomoyasu, Y.; Watanabe, M. et al. (2009). Association of the growth hormone receptor gene polymorphisms with mandibular height in a Korean population. *Arch Oral Biol*, Vol. 54, No. 6, pp. 556-562, ISSN 1879-1506

Kjaer I. (1995). Morphological characteristics of dentitions developing excessive root resorption during orthodontics treatment. *Eur J Orthod*, Vol. 17, No. 1, pp. 25-34, ISSN 0141-5387

Kjelberg, H.; Beiring, M. & Wikland, KA. (2000). Craniofacial morphology, dental occlusion, tooth eruption, and dental maturity in boys of short stature with or without growth hormone deficiency. *Eur J Oral Sci*, Vol. 108, No. 5, pp. 359-367, ISSN 0909-8836

Li, Q.; Zhang, F.; Li, X. & Chen, F. (2010). Genome scan for locus involved in mandibular prognathism in pedigrees from China. *PLoS One*, Vol. 10, No. 5, pp. e12678, ISSN 1932-6203

Li, Q.; Li, X.; Zhang, F. & Chen, F. (2011). The identification of a novel locus for mandibular prognathism in the Han Chinese population. J Dent Res, Vol. 90, No. 1, pp. 53-57, ISSN 1544-0591

Lewinson, D.; Bialik, GM. & Hochberg, Z. (1994) Differential effects of hypothyroidism on the cartilage and the osteogenic process in the mandibular condyle: recovery by growth hormone and thyroxine. *Endocrinology*, Vol. 135, No. 4, pp. 1504-1510, ISSN 0013-7227

Longmate, JA. (2001). Complexity and power in case-control association studies. *Am J Hum Genet*, Vol. 68, No. 5, pp. 1229-1237, ISSN 0002-9297

McFadden, WM.; Engstrom, C.; Engstrom, H. & Anholm, JM. (1989). A study of the relationship between incisor intrusion and root shortening. *Am J Orthod Dentofacial Orthop*, Vol. 96, No. 5, pp. 390-396, ISSN 0889-5406

Miller, RD.; Phillips, MS.; Jo, I.; Donaldson, MA.; Studebaker, JF. & Addleman, N. et al. (2005). The SNP Consortium Allele Frequency Project. High-density single-nucleotide polymorphism maps of the human genome. *Genomics*, Vol. 86, No. 2, pp. 117-126, ISSN 0888-7543

Miyajima, K.; McNamara, JA Jr.; Kimura, T.; Murata, S. & Iizuka, T. (1996). Craniofacial structure of Japanese and European-American adults with normal occlusions and well-balanced faces. *Am J Orthod Dentofacial Orthop*, Vol. 110, No. 4, pp. 431-438, ISSN 0889-5406

Nishioka, M.; Ioi, H.; Nakata, S.; Nakasima, A. & Counts, A. (2006). Root resorption and immune system factors in the Japanese. *Angle Orthod*, Vol. 76, No. 1, pp. 103-108, ISSN 0003-3219

Ong, G. & Neo, J. (1990). A survey of approximal root concavities in an ethnic Chinese population. *Arch Oral Biol*, Vol. 35, No. 11, pp. 925-928, ISSN 0003-9969

Pantel, J.; Machinis, K.; Sobrier, ML.; Duquesnoy, P.; Goosens, M. & Amselem, S. (2000). Species-specific alternative splice mimicry atthe growth hormone receptor locus revealed by the lineage of retroelements during primate evolution. *J Biol Chem*, Vol. 275, No. 25, pp. 18664-18669, ISSN 0021-9258

Pirinen, S.; Majurin, A.; Lenko, HL. & Koski K. (1994). Craniofacial features in patients with deficient and excessive growth hormone. *J Craniofac Genet Dev Biol*, Vol. 14, No. 3, pp. 144-152, ISSN 0270-4145

Pociot, F.; Mølvig, J.; Wogensen, L.; Worsaae, H. & Nerup, J. (1992). A TaqI polymorphism in the human interleukin-1 beta (IL-1 beta) gene correlates with IL-1 beta secretion in vitro. *Eur J Clin Invest*, Vol. 22, No. 6, pp. 396-402, ISSN 0014-2972

Ramirez-Yanez, GO.; Smid, JR.; Young, WG. & Waters, MJ. (2005). Influence of growth hormone on the craniofacial complex of transgenic mice. *Eur J Orthod*, Vol. 27, No. 5, pp. 494-500, ISSN 0141-5387

Roeder, K.; Bacanu, SA.; Wasserman, L. & Devlin, B. (2006). Using linkage genome scans to improve power of association in genome scans. *Am J Hum Genet*, Vol. 78, No. 2, pp. 243-252, ISSN 0002-9297

Rongen-Westerlaken, C.; Vd Born, E.; Prahl-Andersen, B.; Von Teunenbroek, A.; Manesse, P.; Otten, BJ. et al. (1993). Effect of growth hormone treatment on craniofacial growth in Turner's syndrome. *Act Paediatric*, Vol. 82, No. 4, pp. 364–368, ISSN 0803-5253

Sameshima, G.T. & Asgarifar, KO. (2001). Assessment of root resorption and root shape: periapical vs panoramic films, *Angle Orthod*, Vol. 71, No. 3, pp. 185–189, ISSN 0003-3219

Sameshima, GT. & Sinclair, PM. (2001). Predicting and preventing root resorption: Part I. Diagnostic factors. *Am J Orthod Dentofacial Orthop*, Vol. 119, No. 5, pp. 505-510, ISSN 0889-5406

Sanchez, JE.; Perera, E.; Baumbach, L. & Cleveland, WW. (1998). Growth hormone receptor mutations in children with idiopathic short stature. *J Clin Endocrinol Metab*, Vol. 83, No. 11, pp. 4079-4083, ISSN 0021-972X

Sasaki, Y.; Kaida, C.; Saitoh, I.; Fujiwara, T. & Nonaka, K. (2007). Craniofacial growth and functional change in oligodontia with ectodermal dysplasia: a case report. *J Oral Rehabil*, Vol. 34, No. 3, pp. 228-235, ISSN 0305-182X

Sasaki, Y.; Satoh, K.; Hayasaki, H.; Fukumoto, S.; Fujiwara, T. & Nonaka, K. (2009). The P561T polymorphism of the growth hormone receptor gene has an inhibitory effect on mandibular growth in young children. *Eur J Orthod*, Vol. 31, No. 5, pp. 536-541, ISSN 1460-2210

Schaefer, GB.; Rosenbloom, AL.; Guevara-Aguirre, J.; Campbell, EA.; Ullrich, F.; Patil, K. et al. (1994). Facial morphometry of Ecuadorian patients with growth hormone receptor deficiency/Laron syndrome. *J Med Genet*, Vol. 31, No. 8, pp. 635-639, ISSN 0022-2593

Schork, NJ. (2002). Power calculations for genetic association studies using estimated probability distributions. *Am J Hum Genet*, Vol. 70, No. 6, pp. 1480-1489, ISSN 0002-9297

Shevah, O.; Rubinstein, M. & Laron, Z. (2004). Molecular defects of the growth hormone receptor gene, including a new mutation, in Laron syndrome patients in Israel: relationship between defects and ethnic groups. *Isr Med Assoc J*, Vol. 6, No. 10, pp. 630-633, ISSN 1565-1088

Simmons, KE. (1999). Growth hormone and craniofacial changes: preliminary data from studies in Turner's syndrome. *Pediatrics*, Vol. 104, No. 4, pp. 1021-1024, ISSN 0031-4005

Sjoberg, M.; Salazar, T.; Espinosa, C.; Dagnino, A.; Avila, A.; Eggers, M. et al. (2001). Study of GH sensitivity in chilean patients with idiopathic short stature. *J Clin Endocrinol Metab*, Vol. 86, No. 9, PP. 4375-4381, ISSN 0021-972X

Sjogren, K.; Bohlooly, YM.; Olsson, B.; Coschigano, K.; Tornell, J.; Mohan, S. et al. (2000). Disproportional skeletal growth and markedly decreased bone mineral content in growth hormone receptor –/– mice. Biochem Biophys Res Commun, Vol. 267, No. 2, pp. 603-608, ISSN 0006-291X

Tomoyasu Y.; Yamaguchi T.; Tajima A.; Nakajima T.; Inoue I. & Maki K. (2009a). External apical root resorption and interleukin-1B gene polymorphism in Japanese population. *Orthod Waves*, Vol. 68, No. 4, pp. 152-157, ISSN 1344-0241

Tomoyasu, Y.; Yamaguchi, T.; Tajima, A.; Nakajima, T.; Inoue, I. & Maki K. (2009b). Further evidence for an association between mandibular height and the growth hormone receptor gene in a Japanese population. *Am J Orthod Dentofacial Orthop*, Vol. 136, No. 4, pp. 536-541, ISSN 1097-6752

Uematsu, S.; Mogi, M. & Deguchi, T. (1996). Interleukin (IL)-1 beta, IL-6, tumor necrosis factor-alpha, epidermal growth factor, and beta 2-microglobulin levels are elevated in gingival crevicular fluid during human orthodontic tooth movement. *J Dent Res*, Vol. 75, No. 1, pp. 562-567, ISSN 0022-0345

Urbanek, M.; MacLeod, JN.; Cooke, NE. & Liebhaber SA. (1992). Expression of a human growth hormone (hGH) receptor isoform is predicted by tissue-specific alternative splicing of exon 3 of the hGH receptor gene transcript. *Mol Endocrinol*, Vol. 6, No. 2, pp. 279-287, ISSN 0888-8809

Van Erum, R.; Mulier, G.; Carels, C. & de Zegher, F. (1988). Craniofacial growth and dental maturation in short children born small for gestational age: effect of growth hormone treatment. Own observations and review of the literature. *Horm Res*, Vol. 50, No. 3, pp. 141-146, ISSN 0301-0163

Viecilli, RF.; Katona, TR.; Chen, J.; Hartsfield, JK Jr. & Roberts, WE. (2009). Orthodontic mechanotransduction and the role of the P2X7 receptor. *Am J Orthod Dentofacial Orthop*, Vol. 135, No. 6, pp. 694e1–16, ISSN 1097-6752

Wang, XD.; Deng, XY.; Chen, J.; Li, JL.; Chen, X.; Zhao, LZ. et al. (2008). Single nucleotide polymorphisms of the pregnane x receptor gene in Han Chinese and a comparison with other ethnic populations. *Pharmacology*, Vol. 81, No. 4, pp. 350-354, ISSN 1423-0313

Xue, F.; Wong, R. & Rabie, AB. (2010). Identification of SNP markers on 1p36 and association analysis of EPB41 with mandibular prognathism in a Chinese population. *Arch Oral Biol*, Vol. 55, No. 11, pp. 867-872, ISSN 1879-1506

Yamaguchi, T.; Maki, K. & Shibasaki, Y. (2001). Growth hormone receptor gene variant and mandibular height in the normal Japanese population. *Am J Orthod Dentofacial Orthop*, Vol. 119, No. 6, pp. 650-653, ISSN 0889-5406

Yamaguchi, T.; Park, SB.; Narita, A.; Maki, K. & Inoue I. (2005). Genome-wide linkage analysis of mandibular prognathism in Korean and Japanese patients. *J Dent Res*, Vol. 84, No. 3, pp. 255-259, ISSN 0022-0345

Zhou, J.; Lu, Y.; Gao, XH.; Chen, YC.; Lu, JJ.; Bai, YX. et al. (2005). The growth hormone receptor gene is associated with mandibular height in a Chinese population. *J Dent Res*, Vol. 84, No. 11, pp. 1052-1056, ISSN 0022-0345

Permissions

The contributors of this book come from diverse backgrounds, making this book a truly international effort. This book will bring forth new frontiers with its revolutionizing research information and detailed analysis of the nascent developments around the world.

We would like to thank Silvano Naretto MD, DDS, MSc, for lending his expertise to make the book truly unique. He has played a crucial role in the development of this book. Without his invaluable contribution this book wouldn't have been possible. He has made vital efforts to compile up to date information on the varied aspects of this subject to make this book a valuable addition to the collection of many professionals and students.

This book was conceptualized with the vision of imparting up-to-date information and advanced data in this field. To ensure the same, a matchless editorial board was set up. Every individual on the board went through rigorous rounds of assessment to prove their worth. After which they invested a large part of their time researching and compiling the most relevant data for our readers. Conferences and sessions were held from time to time between the editorial board and the contributing authors to present the data in the most comprehensible form. The editorial team has worked tirelessly to provide valuable and valid information to help people across the globe.

Every chapter published in this book has been scrutinized by our experts. Their significance has been extensively debated. The topics covered herein carry significant findings which will fuel the growth of the discipline. They may even be implemented as practical applications or may be referred to as a beginning point for another development. Chapters in this book were first published by InTech; hereby published with permission under the Creative Commons Attribution License or equivalent.

The editorial board has been involved in producing this book since its inception. They have spent rigorous hours researching and exploring the diverse topics which have resulted in the successful publishing of this book. They have passed on their knowledge of decades through this book. To expedite this challenging task, the publisher supported the team at every step. A small team of assistant editors was also appointed to further simplify the editing procedure and attain best results for the readers.

Our editorial team has been hand-picked from every corner of the world. Their multi-ethnicity adds dynamic inputs to the discussions which result in innovative outcomes. These outcomes are then further discussed with the researchers and contributors who give their valuable feedback and opinion regarding the same. The feedback is then collaborated with the researches and they are edited in a comprehensive manner to aid the understanding of the subject.

Apart from the editorial board, the designing team has also invested a significant amount of their time in understanding the subject and creating the most relevant covers. They scrutinized every image to scout for the most suitable representation of the subject and create an appropriate cover for the book.

The publishing team has been involved in this book since its early stages. They were actively engaged in every process, be it collecting the data, connecting with the contributors or procuring relevant information. The team has been an ardent support to the editorial, designing and production team. Their endless efforts to recruit the best for this project, has resulted in the accomplishment of this book. They are a veteran in the field of academics and their pool of knowledge is as vast as their experience in printing. Their expertise and guidance has proved useful at every step. Their uncompromising quality standards have made this book an exceptional effort. Their encouragement from time to time has been an inspiration for everyone.

The publisher and the editorial board hope that this book will prove to be a valuable piece of knowledge for researchers, students, practitioners and scholars across the globe.

List of Contributors

Giampietro Farronato, Cinzia Maspero, Lucia Giannini and Guido Galbiati
Fondazione IRCCS Ca' Granda, Ospedale Maggiore Policlinico, Milan, Italy

Nikolaos Topouzelis
Aristotle University of Thessaloniki, Dental School, Greece

Lisen Espeland and Arild Stenvik
University of Oslo, Norway

Paolo Ronchi
Maxillo-Facial Unit, St. Anna Hospital, Como, Italy

Alberto Guariglia
Private Practice, Milan, Italy

Hicham Khayat
Maitrise Universitaire en Orthodontie et Orthopédie Dento-Faciale, Diplôme Universitaire de Prothèse et de Réhabilitation Maxillo-Faciale, Diplôme Universitaire d'Implantologie Chirurgicale Orale et Maxillo-Faciale, Certificat post-universitaire de Radiologie Tridimensionnelle Dento-Maxillo-Faciale, Head of Polyclinique Dentaire Casablanca's Global care department, Morocco

John K. Neubert, Robert M. Caudle, Calogero Dolce, Edgardo J. Toro, Yvonne Bokrand-Donatelli and L. Shannon Holliday
University of Florida College of Dentistry, United States of America

Kazem Bahaa
Mechatronics Eng. Dept., Baghdad University, Iraq

Garma Noor
Orthodontic Dept., Dentistry College, Baghdad University, Iraq

Yousif Yousif
Ministry of Higher Education and Scientific Research/ R&D Department, Baghdad, Iraq

Bong-Kuen Cha
Gangneung-Wonju National University, Korea

Yoko Tomoyasu, Tetsutaro Yamaguchi and Koutaro Maki
Department of Orthodontics, School of Dentistry, Showa University, Japan